Training Nutrition

The Diet and Nutrition Guide for Peak Performance

Edmund R. Burke, Ph.D.
Jacqueline R. Berning, Ph.D., R.D.

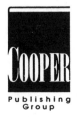
COOPER
Publishing
Group

Library of Congress Cataloging in Publication Data:

Burke, Edmund R., 1949-

TRAINING NUTRITION

Publisher: I. L. Cooper

Library of Congress Catalog Card Number: 92-53280
ISBN: 1-884125-22-0

Printed in the United States of America by Cooper Publishing Group LLC, P.O. Box 562, Carmel, IN 46032.

10 9 8 7 6 5 4 3

The Publisher disclaims responsibility for any adverse effects or consequences from the misapplication or injudicious use of the information contained within this text.

Contents

Foreword

If there is an area in training for athlete performance that is filled with misconceptions, bad information, old wives' tales, and commercial exploitations, it is in determining what to eat to make you a better athlete. We are always seeking a short cut or an easier way. I've grown up through lots of different rules about eating: no water at practice; steak, honey and dry toast for a pre-meal; and now pasta or pancakes. Goodness knows what would have happened if I'd had milk to drink before a ball game or a swimming meet!

Now we have a no-nonsense guide to what is best for us to use as fuel for our bodies. Not just for pre-event eating, but even more specifically for endurance training, speed training, and even for after training and competition . . . who would ever have thought of that! This is not only good science from a highly qualified sports physiologist with a lot of practical experience, but nutritional science from a sports nutritionist with similar experiences. The combination of these two experts and their no nonsense, real world approach to coaches' and athletes' needs fills a real void in our library of training information.

Ray Essick
United States Swimming

Introduction

Athletes, from weekend 5-kilometer runners to million dollar sport stars, all need to be concerned about their diet. Although many of us are meticulous about our training programs, we are often blasé about the need to fuel our bodies for peak performance and training. But to do our best — and to stay healthy and injury free — a balanced diet is also important. A sound diet and the use of specific nutrients, supplements and nutritional ergogenic aids are an integral part of a carefully crafted dietary program.

Optimal nutrition is an integral part of peak performance and can enhance your health and athletic potential, and an inadequate diet and lack of key nutrients can limit your potential for maximum performance.

Interest in sports nutrition is high, but adequate and up-to-date information concerning optimal nutrition is lacking in the sports and fitness arena. What is optimal nutrition and how can you achieve it? Because of the varying requirements in various sports, your optimal diet calls not only for practical experience and individual experimentation but also your knowledge of the basic fundamentals of nutrition. The body's nutrient needs must be considered in view of current findings from physiological, medical, and nutritional research to ascertain the true beneficial effect of nutrition on peak performance both during exercise and in your daily activities.

Certain types of dietary planning do offer a hope for eventual improvement of sports performance. But, it would be foolish to rely too heavily on it, because food and sports supplements are not guaranteed to make you a winner. They are the fuel that powers training, which in turn is the basis for competition. A minimum amount of fuel types are necessary before the process can begin in earnest. But once these minimums are met and exercise is underway, the use of proper nutrition offers no substitute for hard work. It merely promotes hard work and is an insurance policy that opens the door to success.

Most exercising individuals know and listen to their bodies. The underlying philosophy of this book is that understanding how your body uses fuels and what type of fuel is used at rest and during various intensities of exercise can help you perform at your maximum. Whether that maximum is an Olympic event or participating in an amateur sport, the recommendations in this book will benefit anyone at any physical fitness level. Following our suggestions will help you feel better and have more energy when you exercise.

We also believe that individuals who maintain a healthy lifestyle of exercise and wise food choices will not only feel better while participating in exercise, but will establish healthy eating habits that they can follow for the rest of their lives. It is well established that participating in regular exercise and making wise food choices can add more life to your years. We know that teaching and learning comes in many styles.

One teaching style we chose was to use stories about real athletes that we have worked with. Many of their frustrations about training and eating are the same as yours. Their stories and how their fueling problems were solved will help everyone training on a regular basis.

HOW TO USE THIS BOOK

Start at the beginning of this book and work progressively through Chapters 1 to 8. Specifically focus on these main points from each chapter.

Chapter 1. Energy: The Key to Athletic Performance

Chapter One includes basic exercise physiology to explain how your body makes and uses fuels for different levels of exercise. Reading this chapter will assure you of the basic philosophy and knowledge needed to use the rest of the book effectively. Even if you have a general knowledge of exercise, it won't hurt to review the fundamentals.

Chapter 2. Fuel for Endurance Training

This chapter focuses upon what type of fuels the body uses for exercise. You will learn to maximize your muscle glycogen content and what foods will help with endurance. Just as your car cannot perform with diesel gasoline neither can your body. The daily meal plans and sample menus will help you understand that carbohydrates are the super unleaded fuel that your tank needs to feel good and extend your training.

Chapter 3. Competition Nutrition

Putting it all together. Many other sports nutrition books have failed because they always have exercise and eating in separate chapters. Our goal was to put everything about competition nutrition in one chapter, thus easier and more applicable to your training. In this chapter you will learn about pre-event nutrition, eating during the competition, recovery nutrition, and everything in between. You do not have to go to separate chapters on any of these points. We also added recommendations on such topics as fluid replacement before, during and after; carbo-loading before, during and after exercise; as well as fast track snacking.

Chapter 4. Basic Nutrition for Good Health and Performance

While we put everything you wanted to know about training nutrition in Chapter 3, we did feel that if you would like to know more about basic nutrition and healthy eating the opportunity is here in Chapter 4. You can fuel your body properly and still not have a healthy diet. Gaining knowledge on how to make wise food choices from proteins, fats, carbohydrates, vitamins, and minerals will allow you to train and maintain health. Use the diet planning guide at the end of the chapter to assist you in getting all the 40 nutrients you need every day, for health and training.

Chapter 5. Vitamins and Minerals: Team Players

We felt that this chapter and the next (Chapter 6) were essential for the book, simply because of all the misinformation that exists on vitamins and minerals and nutritional ergogenic aids. This chapter is a primer on vitamin and mineral nutrition. It is not meant to answer all the questions about supplements or supplementation but a guide to offer an incentive to learn about the effects of consuming too much of a good thing. Understanding the role of vitamins and minerals in exercise performance permits you to maximize your athletic ability and the opportunity to perform at your best.

Chapter 6. Nutritional Ergogenic Aids

We can't tell you how many times we have been told by athletes (many of them professional or gold medal status) that they have found the secret to maximizing their performance. In many cases these secrets were nutritional ergogenic aids that did nothing but give the athlete a sense that they had some boost in energy or an increased capacity to train. The area of nutritional ergogenic aids is overwhelming, and we chose to put a few of the latest supplements in this chapter. Of particular interest is the latest information on creatine. While the scientific results are encouraging, some practical field testing needs to be done to prove the claims.

Chapter 7. Weight Control

There are millions of books written on this subject and the topic of weight control is a billion dollar industry. What sets this chapter apart from others is that we discuss weight control in the context of an exercising individual. The chapter starts off with body composition rather than focusing on actual weight. There are several body composition techniques discussed in the chapter, and the charts and tables provided in the chapter can help you figure your body composition. If after assessing your body composition you find out that you need to lose some body fat, use the recommendations on proper weight loss techniques. Eating disorders are also discussed because the authors felt that this is a very big problem among active individuals, both males and females. This chapter is also different than other books because it discusses weight management during tapers and off seasons. The chapter concludes by discussing weight gain. While weight gain is not a billion dollar industry, it is a million dollar industry if you include all the products on the market claiming that they will help you gain weight. A true story about a football player wanting to gain weight illustrates the misinformation surrounding nutrition and weight gain.

Chapter 8. Eating on the Road

The authors have watched athletes who followed all the proper training techniques, made excellent food choices to fuel their training, and then go on the road to compete only to have everything fall apart due to the eating habits on the road. Use this chapter to make smart choices at restaurants and avoid traveler's diarrhea. Fueling the body at all-day events is also a problem. The chapter gives guidelines and recommendations on how to eat at all-day events so that you don't become dehydrated or run out of fuel. Using the charts in the chapter will allow you to eat anywhere and still be able to fuel the body.

SUMMARY

Use this book with friends. Having your spouse, family, and training friends participating in making wise food choices for exercising is an added bonus. The information in this book can be more easily learned if you can openly discuss some of the content with others.

The uniqueness of this book is that a credible exercise physiologist and a nutritionist wrote the book together, thus putting training and nutrition together instead of as two separate concepts. There are no gimmicks. No magic potions or magic bullet to help you train harder, faster, or longer. Sound sensible practices have been tested with the many athletes that we have dealt with over the years and are now passing on to you. Your willingness to commit to these suggestions and practices will help you obtain the results you want from your training program and will help you establish healthy eating habits for the rest of your lives. It is your responsibility to exercise regularly and make healthy food choices. We can provide you with precise and factual information, however, the responsibility for training and making wise food choices is ultimately yours. We are confident that the information provided can help you perform at your best. Our goal was to show you how. Your goal is to implement the nutrition strategies suggested in the book. GOOD LUCK!

Ed and Jackie

1 Energy: The Key to Athletic Performance

> "It is not the horse that draws the cart, but the oats."
> —*Russian proverb*

INTRODUCTION

As you begin the transition from rest to moderate activity, of walking to the intense effort of sprinting, many changes take place in your body. For example, you are immediately aware of increased breathing rate and heart rate.

Other noticeable results start to take place after hours and weeks of training. You notice that you can swim, run or cycle farther and faster with less effort. Following a hard workout your heart rate returns to resting faster. You experience a feeling of having more "energy" while performing everyday tasks.

All of these changes, both acute and long term (lower resting heart rate, loss of body fat, increased strength), represent just the "tip of the iceberg" as to what changes are taking place physiologically within your body. Underlying these gross changes are a number of small changes taking place at the cellular level. To really understand what is happening within your exercising body, you must go beyond the system level and explore the changes taking place at the cellular level. This knowledge is basic to understanding the changes that take place with training and your diet.

To any athlete the word "energy" has a particular significance. While everyone needs energy to get through every day, you (as someone who exercises for competition or overall fitness) have put yourself in a position of requiring considerably more energy than the average individual. But beyond just the need for more energy, you have specially adapted and developed physiological systems for optimal use and storage of energy.

What substances supply the energy you need? And how are these substances utilized to provide the energy to ride a bicycle, for example, 50 miles? Or to swim for two hours?

The energy requirements to run a marathon may be as high as

1

2600 calories. Twenty-six hundred calories is more than the average sedentary individual will consume in a 24-hour period. When you consider the amount of food that can be taken in during the race in the form of sport drinks and energy bars, it becomes very clear that one must rely heavily on body stores to supply the energy needed to run such an event. **Your body's need for energy is second only to air and water.**

There are three major energy stores in your body; fat (in the form of adipose tissue), carbohydrate (in the form of liver and muscle glycogen), and protein (in the form of muscles and tissue). As you will see later, muscle glycogen is the most important energy stores for prolonged exercise. But, as we will also see, fats and proteins are of significance during exercise.

Before the significance and function of these storage fuels can be understood, you must first comprehend the events that supply and control all energy metabolism.

ATP: THE ENERGY CURRENCY

Body cells use the energy in carbohydrates, fats, and proteins for one major purpose — to continually form adenosine triphosphate, or simply ATP. ATP is the ultimate fuel source for your cells. Water and specific vitamins and minerals are used also in energy production to help your body cells turn the stored energy in food into ATP.

Energy is released in your body when carbohydrates, fats, and proteins are burned inside your cells. But, before you can use the energy in carbohydrates, proteins, and fats these nutrients must be broken down (digested) in your stomach into smaller particles and absorbed in the intestines. Protein breaks down into amino acids, fat into fatty acids and carbohydrate into glucose. These smaller particles are absorbed from your intestine into your bloodstream and transported to your muscle cells. Once they are inside the muscles, they are chemically changed into the energy-rich substance called ATP.

Your body produces ATP — the ultimate energy necessary for training and competition — in two ways: without oxygen (called the anaerobic pathway) and with oxygen (called the aerobic pathway). Both pathways supply energy to your body during exercise. However, usually one pathway is dominant during any specific activity. Table 1.1 lists examples of sports and their predominant metabolic pathway.

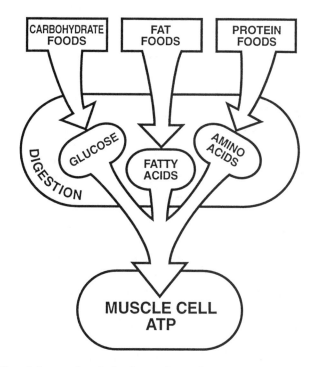

Figure 1.1. Breakdown of carbohydrate, fat and protein for energy production.

Table 1.1. Energy pathways for the production of ATP and predominant sports.

Anaerobic:
Immediate power output, strength training, high intensity, short duration

Sports such as: weight lifting, football, sprinting, gymnastics

Aerobic:
Long-term exercise, endurance training, lower intensity, long duration

Sports such as: cross-country skiing, road cycling, marathon running, hiking

ANAEROBIC PATHWAYS

The ATP-CP Pathway

ATP stores in your muscle cells is very limited. In fact, there is only enough ATP stored in your body to last several seconds of intensive exercise. So ATP must continuously be resynthesized to provide a continuous supply of energy. Creatine phosphate (CP) is a high energy rich compound stored within your muscles, whose chemical bond is similar to ATP and contains a great deal of energy. When CP's chemical bonds are broken, energy is released which can be used to resynthesize ATP. CP is your muscles' high-octane fuel supply to rebuild your ATP stores.

Energy released from the breakdown of ATP and CP will supply your muscles for high-intensity exercise for about five to ten seconds. If you need to continue a high energy output for a few minutes, additional sources of energy must be provided for the resynthesis of ATP.

Anaerobic Glycolysis Pathway

A second metabolic pathway within your muscle cells capable of rapidly producing ATP via the breakdown of carbohydrates anaerobically (without oxygen) is known as glycolysis. The carbohydrate which is stored within your muscle cells is known as glycogen. Glycogen is, simply, a long branched string of glucose (sugar) molecules. Glycolysis involves the breakdown of a single glucose molecule to produce ATP.

The anaerobic glycolytic pathway provides energy for short-duration, high-intensity exercise. This pathway is designed for intense bursts of speed such as sprinting down the basketball court or jumping to spike the ball in volleyball (approximately 10 seconds to several minutes). The anaerobic pathway provides instantaneous energy but cannot provide ATP energy for long periods of time.

One important point to consider during anaerobic work is that only glucose can be used to supply ATP. ATP production during anaerobic metabolism provides a rapid, but limited, form of energy when oxygen supplies are inadequate. In addition, the rapid production of ATP via this pathway has one major drawback: lactic acid.

When you put heavy demands on your glycolytic anaerobic pathway, levels of lactic acid increase quickly in your muscles, which causes fatigue. Regular anaerobic training enables you to work at greater intensities with lower levels of lactic acid. This increase in maximal work intensity is due to an increase in muscular strength and an increased ability to buffer lactic acid. Anaerobic and aerobic training programs can be designed to combine high-intensity and prolonged submaximal exercise to improve the removal of lactic acid and delay fatigue.

The Aerobic Pathway

The aerobic pathway is important during lower-intensity, pro-

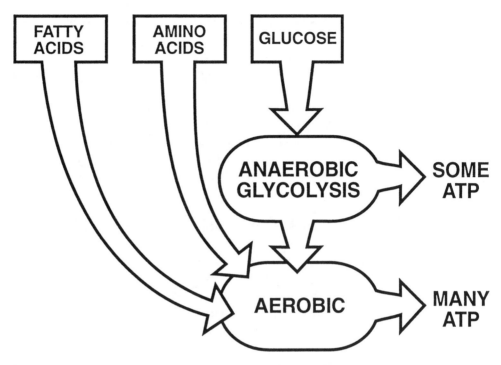

Figure 1.2. Energy production in both anaerobic glycolysis and aerobic pathways.

longed exercise or training. This pathway provides much of the energy for longer term exercise, usually over two to three minutes, in activities such as cross-country skiing, road cycling, swim training and distance running.

In addition to glucose, protein and fat may also be converted to energy in the aerobic pathway. It is important to know that protein and fat cannot produce energy anaerobically; they only provide energy in the aerobic pathway.

When you begin to exercise, you may start out using primarily the anaerobic pathways, and after a few minutes the aerobic pathway begins to take over.

As we have seen, endurance training results in changes to your body. First, there is the increased ability to provide oxygen to your working muscles. This happens by an increase in the number of red blood cells and capillaries (blood vessels) which carry oxygen to your working muscles with a concurrent increase in the energy producing structures called mitochondria within your muscle cells.

When your body burns nutrients for energy, oxygen passes through the mitochondria to furnish energy for muscular contraction. Therefore, regular endurance-aerobic training increases oxygen delivery to the working muscles causing an increased ability for your muscles to produce more energy. The result is that you are able to exercise longer and at a higher intensity than your lesser trained friends.

Training increases the capacities of both the aerobic and anaerobic pathways. Endurance training is primarily aerobic and will increase the circulation of oxygen throughout your body and enhance the oxygen used by the muscles. Anaerobic adaptations to training increase the ability of your body to remove lactic acid from your system as well as increase your muscle size and strength.

DETERMINATION OF EXERCISE FUEL USAGE ———

A variety of factors determine when your muscles use fats, carbohydrates and proteins during exercise. These include: the intensity of the exercise, the duration of the exercise session, the composition of your diet, and your fitness level. Let's explore how each of these factors will affect your performance both in training and competition.

Intensity

The intensity of your effort (percentage of your maximum heart rate) is particularly important in determining your muscle's energy production. Low intensity exercise, like walking or completing a slow warm-up in the pool, is fueled by a slow rate of aerobic ATP production. At rest or during low-intensity exercise, carbohydrates supply about half of your body's energy needs. The other half comes mainly from fat, and a very small amount from protein. As the intensity of exercise increases, ATP production must also go up.

This demand is met mainly by an increase in the rate of anaerobic ATP production from glucose. During heavy fatiguing exercise, like sprinting, ATP must be produced rapidly, therefore, glycogen becomes the predominant fuel source. Moderate-intensity training improves your body cells' ability to burn more fat aerobically at higher intensities of physical activity. Also, hormonal changes take place — increased release of epinephrine and norepinephrine, decreased insulin secretion — which promote the release of fatty acids from your fat stores. This spares your muscle's glycogen stores so your muscle's glucose stores last longer and your endurance improves.

If you want to improve your capacity for moderate intensity exercise, exercise at 50 to 80 percent of maximal aerobic capacity (or 60 to 86 percent of maximum heart rate) in such activities as distance running or swimming. Concentrate on training your aerobic energy pro-

Table 1.2. Exercise intensity and fuel usage.

Exercise Intensity (% max heart rate)	Main Source of Fuel
40-60	Mostly fat stores
60-80	Fat and carbohydrate about evenly
80-90	Mainly carbohydrate
>90	Nearly 100 percent carbohydrate

duction system. This means planning your training to include moderate intensity endurance training several days per week.

On the other hand, if you want to maximize performance for high-intensity activity (above 80 percent of aerobic capacity, or 87 percent of your maximum heart rate) such as sprinting, basketball or soccer, it is important to train your anaerobic energy system. This means incorporating high-intensity work into your weekly program to help build your ATP and CP stores. High-intensity exercise will also help you tolerate higher levels of lactic acid.

If your events combine both low- and high-intensity efforts, you must train both your anaerobic and aerobic energy releasing systems in order to achieve consistent top performances.

Table 1.3. Fuel use during high-intensity exercise. Exercise above 80% of maximum heart rate affects the type of fuel used during exercise.

Increased glucose metabolism:
• supplies ATP rapidly
• increased production of lactic acid
• limited supply in liver and muscle glycogen

Decreased fat metabolism:
• lactic acid impedes the release of fat
• cannot supply ATP rapidly

Exercise Duration

The duration of your physical activity or sport also helps define whether the fuel used for energy production will be carbohydrate, fat or protein. If you spend more time running, cycling or swimming, the more your body will rely upon more fat to be burned as a fuel. Your fat stores will supply as much as 60 to 70 percent of your energy needs for moderate-intensity exercise that last more than four hours.

In events such as the marathon, long distance cycling and cross-country skiing, as the race progresses, intensity usually has to decrease, since your body begins to run out of its limited supply of glycogen. When your glycogen stores are low, fat metabolism supplies most of the energy needed for exercise, along with a small amount of protein. But, remember fat can only be used up to 60 to 70 percent of your aerobic capacity.

Protein should be thought of as a "back-up" fuel. When carbohydrate stores are low, or during prolonged exercise, protein breakdown may be enhanced, but it is incorrect to think of protein as a major fuel source, or to eat large protein meals in an effort to increase energy output. The principle role of protein is to build muscle tissue, hormones, and antibodies as well as other important functions. Providing a back-up fuel source is a secondary role of the protein you eat.

For most athletes it must be noted that muscle glycogen and glucose supplied from your bloodstream is the predominant fuel for exercise up to about 90 minutes. It takes about 20 minutes for fat to be mobilized into fatty acids from your fat stores.

Table 1.4. Examples of events competed at maximum effort and the type of fuel usage.

Event	Percent of Maximum Heart Rate	Glycogen Contribution	Fat Contribution
Marathon	70-95%	70%	30%
Half-marathon	80-95%	70%	30%
400-meter Sprint	100%	100%	0%

Diet

Another factor that influences the fuels burned during exercise is diet. The amount of fat and carbohydrate you consume in your diet will also determine the amount of fat and glycogen used as fuel during competition. If your diet is high in fat, your body will tend to use more fat as a fuel. If your diet is high in carbohydrate, your body will burn more glycogen for energy. Eating a high-carbohydrate diet (60-65 percent of caloric intake) will allow for a greater utilization of glycogen. A high-fat, low-carbohydrate diet (<35 percent of calories as fat) will promote the use of fat as a fuel in your body.

It is not recommended that trained, exercising individuals switch to a high-fat diet. Even the leanest athletes have more fat stored than they could possibly use during an endurance event. For example, a lean runner has enough fat stores to run from San Francisco to Los Angeles. However, their carbohydrate stores will only last about the first 25 miles. Now you may be thinking, "What's the problem? Since I have plenty of fat stores, I don't have to worry about carbohydrate; I'll just run the distance on my fat stores." Unfortunately, your body does not work that way. Some carbohydrate is needed to burn fat. Carbohydrate must be present to serve as a primer in order to burn fat as a fuel. Think of fat as the wood you put in the fireplace, and carbohydrate as the ignition fuel. You may have enough wood to heat your house for one month, but if you don't have matches, you'll never get the fire started.

Lastly, high-fat diets lower muscle glycogen stores, which we now know will reduce your ability to sustain high-intensity exercise. Low-muscle glycogen stores will also limit your endurance capacity. Thus, it is critical to consume a minimum of 60 percent of your calories as carbohydrates to ensure optimal glycogen stores in your muscles.

Your Fitness Level

The last factor that determines what fuel the body will burn is fitness level. When you are in shape, the body becomes more efficient at producing energy aerobically at the same absolute intensity of effort. For example, after a few months of training you will be able to work at a lower percentage of your maximum aerobic capacity while running, cycling or swimming at the same pace or speed. This is good news to your muscle fuel stores. Now, you will be able to use more fat and less glycogen at the same absolute level of exercise.

When just starting an exercise program, untrained individuals begin to accumulate lactic acid in their muscles around 50 to 60 percent of their maximal aerobic capacity. Trained athletes do not begin to accumulate lactic acid until about 70 to 75 percent of their maximal capacity. Most often this intensity is referred to as "anaerobic" or "lactate" threshold, and sport scientists like to report this value as a percentage of one's maximal aerobic capacity.

The fitter you are, the better your muscles will use fat as the main

Table 1.5. Benefits of increased levels of physical fitness.

- Increased ability of the muscles to use fat as a fuel source during aerobic exercise

- Increased muscle stores of glycogen

- During endurance exercise, glycogen stores are used more slowly, "sparing muscle glycogen" for increased exercise performance

- Lactic acid begins to accumulate at a higher aerobic intensity, impedes the use of fat as a fuel and increases muscle glycogen use

- Increased fitness allows for better weight control, since fat is more readily burned during exercise.

fuel source for aerobic energy production. When you burn more fat, less stored muscle glycogen is used during exercise. In the sports nutrition world this is known as "glycogen sparing" and plays an important role in your ability to exercise for extended periods of time.

Lastly, training allows your muscles to store more glycogen. Trained athletes are able to store about 50 percent more glycogen than an untrained individual. The good news is that increasing your fitness level allows you to store more glycogen and use more fat during exercise to spare glycogen for higher intensity efforts.

PULLING IT ALL TOGETHER

Utilizing fat, carbohydrate or protein to provide ATP during exercise is not like turning the dial on your radio. That is, it is rare that you use only fat and "turn off" carbohydrate and protein, or visa versa — these are all used together. However, anaerobic activity is another story. When you work near or at maximal intensities, carbohydrate is the only fuel you can use. During prolonged physical activity, such as cycling, triathlons and long-distance swimming, the amounts of fat, carbohydrate and protein that is used may transiently rise and fall, depending upon the duration and intensity of the activity, the food and drink you eat prior to and during exercise, how fit you are, and various other factors that we will discuss in later chapters.

2 Fuel for Endurance Training

"Evander Holyfield's got a nutritionist, and I've got room service."
—*George Foreman*

INTRODUCTION

Mary was returning to hard training after one week off from basketball practice due to an injury, but after several days she found that she could not make it through 90 minutes of hard practice without feeling totally fatigued. John is preparing for his first half-marathon. During his final weeks of hard training, he finds that after two or three days of hard mileage, he cannot seem to recover properly for the next day's training sessions.

Both individuals, while having enough fat stores to perform unbelievable endurance events, are about to find out that it's their carbohydrate stores that limited their ability to train intensely.

A nutritional concern for most individuals exercising daily is consuming enough carbohydrate. No matter how well conditioned these athletes are, glycogen (which is stored on a limited basis) is used as a major fuel source during moderate to high-intensity exercise. If daily carbohydrate intake is not enough to replace the muscle glycogen used during training, muscle glycogen levels drop and the athlete does not have enough fuel to train properly. Even the best conditioned athletes can experience reduced performance and fatigue if muscle glycogen levels are below normal during periods of hard training. The same holds true for competition as we will see in a later chapter.

The "staleness" and general feeling of "overtraining" that you may experience during hard training may be partially due to a reduction in muscle glycogen and may be brought about by not eating enough foods high in carbohydrate. This "chronic fatigue" often keeps you from maintaining a proper training schedule and ultimately will keep you from competing at your maximal capacity.

The carbohydrate stores of an active 150-pound man total about 1,800 calories. Of these, 1,400 calories are in the muscles, where they can be used directly; 320 calories are in the liver, where they can be released into the bloodstream; and about 80 calories are in the blood, and can travel to where they are needed (including the brain, which

11

can only burn glucose). While these numbers may seem large, they will last only about two hours during high-intensity exercise.

STRESSING YOUR GLYCOGEN STORES

As early as the 1930's, scientists observed that endurance activities could be improved by increasing carbohydrates in one's diet. A diet rich in carbohydrates increases endurance capabilities because increased stores of glycogen in the muscles will reduce fatigue during prolonged exercise.

In one series of experiments, subjects consumed three different diets and then rode a bicycle ergometer to exhaustion. All diets maintained normal caloric intake but in the first diet most of the calories were consumed in the form of fat. The second diet was a mixed diet of carbohydrates, proteins and fats, with carbohydrates comprising about 50 percent of the total calories. The third diet was over 70 percent carbohydrates. The results shown in Figure 2.1 clearly point to the fact that leg muscles of the subjects, when fed a high-carbohydrate diet, had the greatest endurance capacity.

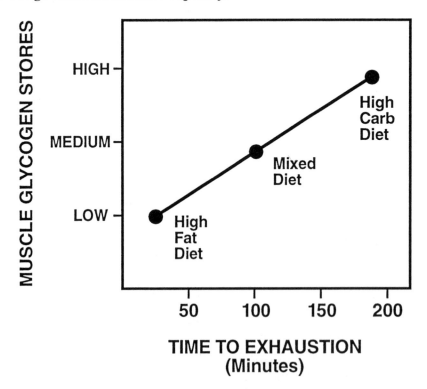

Figure 2.1. Effects of various diets on time to exhaustion while exercising.

Work completed in the early 1980's by Dr. David Costill showed that if athletes did not consume a diet adequately high in carbohydrates on a daily basis, they would experience chronic depletion of glycogen and fatigue, as shown in Figure 2.2. This is the situation experienced by many athletes in hard training who do not consume adequate carbohydrate on a daily basis.

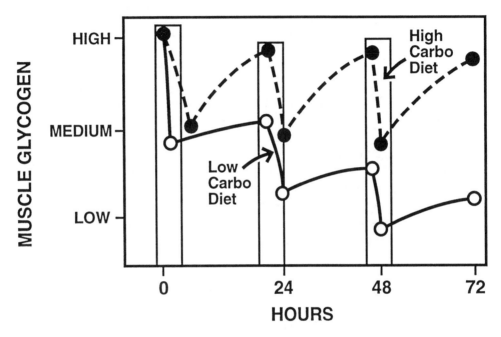

Figure 2.2. High-carbohydrate diet speeds recovery after training.

PROPER DAILY FUEL MIX

Your daily energy needs will depend both upon the duration and intensity of your training program. Many athletes train intensely for over 90 minutes per day and expend from 1000 to 1400 calories during this time. A 150-pound athlete exercising this hard will need to consume about 3,500 calories per day to stay in energy balance.

Also, this athlete will need to eat a healthy mix of foods to ensure proper energy levels of the three major food fuel sources. A diet of 60 percent carbohydrate, 25 percent fat and 15 percent protein, with an adequate amount of calories geared to your activity level, is needed on a daily basis. Whether you are wanting to lose, gain or maintain a steady weight, you need to strive to maintain the above ratios.

The above athlete will have to consume 525 grams of carbohydrates (2,100 calories) to reach his goal of 60 percent. First, you multiply the number of calories you take in daily by the percentage of carbohydrate calories needed (60 percent). This figure gives you the number of carbohydrate calories you need. In the above example, 3,500 calories times 60 percent equals 2,100 calories. Then you need to divide the 2,100 calories by 4 (carbohydrates provide 4 calories per gram) to get the number of carbohydrate grams needed, or 525 grams.

Reading Labels

Now you have to learn how to read labels. After you have calculated the number of grams of carbohydrate you need read the labels of all the food you eat to see how many grams of carbohydrate you are consuming. See how it compares to the 60 percent level required for proper nutritional performance. Refer to Appendix C for tips on reading labels.

We should mention that while most athletes recognize the need for more carbohydrate in their diet, their diets often contain less than 50 percent carbohydrate. As we have mentioned, this may be the primary reason why they feel chronically fatigued and stale during periods of intense training.

THE NUTRITIOUS GAME PLAN ⸻⸻⸻⸻

Most of us think of bread and pasta as the only good sources of carbohydrates. However, an apple, glass of juice, candy bar and energy drinks also contain carbohydrates.

Remember that carbohydrates come in several forms — complex and simple carbohydrates, and a combination of the two. Starches (such as rice, pasta, breads, cereals and vegetables) are good sources of complex carbohydrates. Fructose (found in fruit and fruit juices), sucrose (table sugar), glucose and lactose (found in milk) are examples of simple carbohydrates. Mixed carbohydrates (such as in candy bars, cookies and cakes) contain both simple and complex carbohydrates.

You can often obtain additional carbohydrates in your diet by eating more bread, cereal, rice and pasta at mealtime, or some raisins, candy or cookies as a convenient snack.

Table 2.1 contains a listing of the carbohydrate content of various foods available to you while training on a daily basis. If you want more information on the nutrient and caloric content of foods, talk to a registered dietitian or exercise scientist. You may also want to consult

Table 2.1. Selected high-carbohydrate foods. Foods that can be used both for the pre-exercise meal and for post-exercise.

Food	Calories	Carbohydrate (grams)	Fat (grams)
Apple, medium	81	21	0
Grapes, 1 cup	58	16	0
Strawberry yogurt, 1 cup	257	43	3.5
Applesauce, ½ cup	97	26	0
Banana, medium	105	27	0
Baked potato, large	139	32	0
Raisins, ⅔ cup	300	78	0
Whole wheat bread, 1 slice	61	11	1
Noodles, egg, 1 cup	178	33	2
White toast, 1 slice	64	12	1
Spaghetti, 1 cup	179	34	1.5
Rice, 1 cup	205	45	0
Cornbread, 1 piece	198	29	7
Kellogg's Frosted Pop Tart	200	38	5
Jelly, grape, 1 tbsp.	50	13	0
Fig Newtons, 2 cookies	100	20	0
Bagel, medium	163	31	1
Pancakes 3 (4 in.)	260	51	3

Bowes and Church's Food Values of Portions Commonly Used, published by Pennington and Church, Philadelphia, J. B. Lippincott, Co., 1989.

Beware of Foods Believed to Be High in Carbohydrates

During many of our training camps at the Olympic Training Center, we are amazed at how many athletes do not know how to recognize foods high in "carbo's." Many athletes are surprised to discover that foods they thought were high in carbohydrate are actually high in fat. You can use the information from food labels to help calculate the percentage of carbohydrates in the particular can or box of food you are eating. Here is a simple method for making that conversion: Multiply the number of grams of carbohydrate per serving by four. This gives you the total number of carbohydrate calories per serving. Next, divide the number of carbohydrate calories by the total number of calories per serving to get the percentage of carbohydrate calories per serving.

An example would be a chocolate croissant eaten by a swimmer for breakfast which has 25 grams of carbohydrate per serving and 260 calories per croissant (one serving). 100 calories of carbohydrate in 260 calories equals only 38 percent carbohydrate. In fact, this croissant is

60 percent fat, not 60 percent carbohydrate. You will be surprised by how many supposedly high-carbohydrate foods are really high-fat foods.

Because not all high-carbohydrate foods are labeled, Table 2.2 will give you an idea of foods you should be selecting to ensure adequate carbohydrate intake.

Table 2.2. Guide for selecting low-fat foods.

	Select	Use Moderately	Avoid
Grains			
Bread	Whole grain bread Bagel English muffin Pita bread	Pancake Hamburger bun Bran muffin Taco shell	Doughnut French toast Pastry Croissants
Cereals	Whole grain cereals	Instant cereals	Granola
Rice/Pasta	Plain rice Plain pasta		Fried rice Pasta/Cream sauce
Fruits and Vegetables			
Fruits	Dried fruit Fresh, frozen, or canned fruit Fruit salad with low-fat yogurt		Fruit salad with whip cream
Vegetables	Fresh, frozen or canned Potatoes (baked, boiled) Mashed potatoes (made with skim milk)	Avocados Mashed potatoes (made with whole milk)	Creamed vegetables Potatoes (fried, au gratin, creamed) Deep fried vegetables
Snacks			
	Pretzels Air popped popcorn Rice cakes Soda crackers Graham crackers	Reduced-fat party mix Oil popped popcorn Bread sticks with cheese	Regular party mix Oil popped popcorn with butter Microwave popcorn Potato, corn chips Snack crackers
Dairy Products			
Milk	Skim or 1% milk Buttermilk	2% milk 4% fat cottage cheese	Whole milk Creamed cottage cheese
Cheese	1% cottage cheese Mozzarella cheese Parmesan cheese Ricotta cheese	Neufchatel cheese Farmers cheese Processed cheese food	Cheddar, colby cheese American cheese Swiss cheese Brick, Monterey jack
Yogurt	Non-fat yogurt Fat-free frozen dessert Fat-free frozen yogurt Skim-milk pudding	2-4% fat yogurt Ice milk Low-fat frozen yogurt 2% milk pudding	Whole milk yogurt Ice cream Milkshake (whole milk) Whole-milk pudding

Table 2.2. (*Continued*)

	Select	Use Moderately	Avoid
Protein Foods			
Meat	Flank steak Sirloin Veal Venison	Beef stew Hamburger (80% lean) Pork Ham (roasted, canned)	Liver, giblets Ribs (baked, boiled) Canned meat Hamburger (70% lean)
Poultry	Chicken, no skin Turkey, no skin Wild game	Chicken with skin Turkey with skin	Fried chicken Duck or goose
Seafood	Unbreaded fish Fresh or frozen salmon	Oil-packed fish, drained Crab cakes	Deep-fried fish Deep-fried seafood
Eggs	Egg whites Egg substitutes	Whole eggs (boiled)	Whole eggs (fried) Omelets
Cold Cuts	Turkey hot dogs Turkey sausage Deli chicken, turkey	Reduced-fat luncheon meats Sliced, deli meats	Hot dogs Sausage Sliced bologna
Meat Substitutes	Dried beans and peas Vegetables, refried beans Tofu	Canned baked beans Refried beans with lard Natural peanut butter	Beans with pork Processed peanut butter

DAILY MEAL PLANNING

You can control how much and what kind of fuel is in your "tank" by paying attention to what you eat on a daily basis. On the next few pages are sample menus for different energy needs. These are planned menus that are high in carbohydrates and low in fats and proteins to keep you running at peak capacity. Use these menus as guides, and you may adapt and substitute foods as you see fit.

If your caloric needs are high, you may not be able to eat enough food at three meals to get all the calories and carbohydrates you need. If this is the case, supplements and snacks are important. However, these foods should be chosen carefully, because most snack foods are high in fat.

Carbohydrate supplementation is essential to meet the needs of heavy training. Greater portions of pasta, potatoes, and breads can help, but many athletes may prefer the concentrated carbohydrate found in "high-carbohydrate drinks." Such products as Ultra Fuel® (Twinn Laboratories), Exceed High-Carbohydrate Source® (Weider Group) and GatorLode® (Gatorade) are used to generate additional carbohydrate intake without the bulk of solid food. Additional quantities of high-carbohydrate drinks can be easily integrated into your daily menu to supplement normal carbohydrate intake. Similarly, these high-energy drinks can be added to your meals or used as a nutritious, high-carbohydrate snack between meals.

Nutrition is a tool that you have available to you to help improve training and athletic performance. The contribution of carbohydrates to a good training diet can make you a better performer and increase your energy output. Yet, carbohydrate input is so intimately related to work output that the two cannot be considered independent of each other.

Table 2.3. Examples of various high-carbohydrate, low-fat menus (tsp=teaspoon, oz=ounces, T=tablespoons, fl=fluid).

Examples of 2000 Calorie High-Carbohydrate, Low-Fat Menus

Day One:

Breakfast:
>   Scrambled eggs:
>   1 large egg and 2 egg whites cooked in 1 tsp margarine
>   2 slices of whole-wheat toast
>   2 tsp of jelly
>   1 apple

Lunch:
>   1½ cups macaroni
>   2 oz. mozzarella cheese
>   1 carrot
>   1 cup strawberries

Dinner:
>   3 oz of beef tenderloin (broiled)
>   1 medium baked potato
>   3 T low-fat yogurt
>   1 whole-grain dinner roll
>   2 cups of broccoli
>   ½ cup of milk

Snack 1: 8 oz can of liquid sports supplement*

Snack 2: 8 fl oz of high-carbohydrate drink**

Day Two:

Breakfast:
>   ½ cup cooked oatmeal
>   1 cup of skim milk
>   1 blueberry muffin (homemade)
>   2 tsp jelly
>   1 tsp margarine

Table 2.3. *(Continued)*

Lunch:
>Ham sandwich;
>>2 oz ham (boiled)
>>1 tsp mustard
>>1 lettuce leaf
>>2 slices of rye bread
>½ cup peas
>1 cup of skim milk
>½ cantaloupe

Dinner:
>1½ cup of spaghetti/meat sauce:
>>2 oz of ground beef per serving
>Slice of tomato and lettuce
>1 cup skim milk
>½ cup of grapes

Snack 1: 1 cup (8 fl oz) of a metabolic optimizer***

Snack 2: 1 cup (8 fl oz) high-carbohydrate drink

Day Three:

Breakfast:
>1 shredded-wheat biscuit
>1 cup skim milk
>½ English muffin
>1 tsp margarine

Lunch:
>Tuna salad:
>>¼ cup of water-pack tuna
>>1 tsp mayonnaise
>>½ cup lettuce
>>½ cup croutons
>1 hard roll
>1 banana

Dinner:
>1 hamburger
>>3 oz ground round (boiled)
>>1 bun
>>2 tsp catsup
>1 small potato (boiled)
>1 cup carrots
>1 cup skim milk
>½ cup gelatin with fruit

Snack 1: 1 cup (8 fl oz) of a metabolic optimizer

Snack 2: 1 cup (8 fl oz) high-carbohydrate drink

Table 2.3. (*Continued*)

Examples of 3000 Calorie High-Carbohydrate, Low-Fat Menus

Day One:

Breakfast:

    Scrambled eggs:

        1 large egg and 2 egg whites cooked in 1 tsp margarine

    2 slices of whole-wheat toast

    2 tsp of jelly

    1 apple

Lunch:

    1½ cups macaroni/tomato sauce

    1 cup of cream of potato soup

    1 carrot

    1 bran muffin (homemade)

    2 tsp margarine

    1 cup of strawberries

    2 tsp of brown sugar

Dinner:

    3 oz of beef tenderloin (boiled)

    2 medium potatoes (baked)

    3 T low-fat yogurt

    2 whole-grain dinner rolls

    2 tsp margarine

    2 cups broccoli

    1 cup ice milk

Snack 1: 8 oz can of a sports nutritional supplement

Snack 2: 1 cup (8 fl oz) high-carbohydrate drink

Day Two:

Breakfast:

    ½ cup cooked oatmeal

    1 cup skim milk

    1 blueberry muffin (homemade)

    2 tsp margarine

    1, 8 oz can of sports nutritional supplement

Lunch:

    Tomato and cucumber sandwich:

        1 sliced tomato

        6 slices of cucumber

        2 tsp of mayonnaise

        2 slices of white bread

    ½ cup peas

    1 piece of cornbread

    1 cup of skim milk

    ½ cantaloupe

Table 2.3. *(Continued)*

Dinner:
>
> 2½ cups spaghetti/meat sauce:
>> 2 oz ground round beef
>
> Sliced tomato and lettuce
> 3 slices of garlic bread
> 2 tsp of Italian dressing
> 1 cup of skim milk
> ½ cup of grapes

Snack 1: 8 oz of high-carbohydrate energy drink

Snack 2: 8 oz can of sports nutritional supplement

Day Three:

Breakfast:
>
> 1 shredded-wheat biscuit
> 1 cup of skim milk
> ½ English muffin
> 2 tsp of honey
> 1 tsp of margarine
> 1, 8 oz can of a sports nutritional supplement

Lunch:
>
> Cottage cheese and fruit salad:
>> ¼ cup low-fat cottage cheese
>> 2 tsp mayonnaise
>> 1 pear
>
> 2 hard rolls
> 2 tsp margarine
> 1 banana

Dinner:
>
> 1 hamburger:
>> 3 oz ground round (boiled)
>> 1 bun
>> 2 tsp catsup
>
> 2 medium potatoes (baked)
> 1 ear of corn
> 3 tsp margarine
> 1 cup carrots
> 1 cup skim milk
> ½ cup gelatin with fruit

Snack 1: 8 oz can of liquid sports supplement

Snack 2: 8 fl oz of high-carbohydrate drink

Table 2.3. *(Continued)*

Examples of 4000 Calorie High-Carbohydrate, Low-Fat Menus

Day One:

Breakfast:

      Scrambled eggs:

          1 large egg and 2 egg whites cooked in

          1 tsp margarine

      2 slices whole-wheat toast

      2 tsp jelly

      1 apple

      1, 8 oz can of liquid sports nutritional supplement

Lunch:

      2½ cups macaroni/tomato sauce

      1 cup of cream of potato soup

      1 carrot

      2 bran muffins (homemade)

      2 tsp margarine

      1 cup of strawberries

      2 tsp brown sugar

Dinner:

      6 fl oz of grape juice

      3 oz beef tenderloin (boiled)

      2 medium potatoes (baked)

      3 T low-fat yogurt

      2 whole-grain dinner rolls

      2 tsp margarine

      2 cups of broccoli

      1 cup of ice milk

      2 T fudge sauce

Snack 1: 2 cup (16 fl oz) high-carbohydrate drink

Snack 2: 1 cup (8 fl oz) of a metabolic optimizer

Snack 3: 1 can (8 fl oz) of sports nutritional supplement

Day Two:

Breakfast:

      1 shredded-wheat biscuit

      1 cup of skim milk

      ½ English muffin

      2 tsp honey

      1 tsp margarine

      1 can (8 fl oz) sports nutritional supplement

Table 2.3. (*Continued*)

Lunch:
  Cottage cheese and fruit salad:
    ¼ cup low-fat cottage cheese
    2 tsp mayonnaise
    1 pear
  2 hard rolls
  2 tsp margarine
  banana
  1 serving strawberry shortcake

Dinner:
  1 hamburger:
    3 oz ground round (boiled)
    1 bun
    2 tsp catsup
  2 medium potatoes (baked)
  2 ears corn
  4 tsp margarine
  1 cup carrots
  1 cup skim milk
  ½ cup gelatin with fruit

Snack 1: 2 cup (16 fl oz) high-carbohydrate drink

Snack 2: 1 cup (8 fl oz) of a metabolic optimizer

Snack 3: 1 can (8 fl oz) of sports nutritional supplement

Day Three:

Breakfast:
  ½ cup of cooked oatmeal
  1 cup of skim milk
  1 blueberry muffin (homemade)
  2 tsp margarine
  1, 8 oz can of sports nutritional supplement

Lunch:
  Tomato and cucumber sandwich:
    1 sliced tomato
    6 slices of cucumber
    2 tsp mayonnaise
    2 slices of white bread
  ½ cup peas
  2 pieces of cornbread
  1 tsp of margarine
  1 cup skim milk
  ½ cantaloupe

Table 2.3. (*Continued*)

Dinner:

        1 cup grapefruit juice

        3 cups of spaghetti/meat sauce:

            2 oz of ground round per serving

        Sliced tomato and lettuce/2 tsp Italian dressing

        3 slices of garlic bread

        1 cup of skim milk

        ½ cup of grapes

        1 slice of carrot cake

Snack 1: 2 cup (16 fl oz) high-carbohydrate drink

Snack 2: 1 cup (8 fl oz) of a metabolic optimizer

Snack 3: 1 can (8 fl oz) of sports nutritional supplement

---

   * Examples of sports nutritional supplements are: Exceed Sports Nutritional®, Nutriment®, GatorPro®, Sport Shake®

  ** Examples of high-carbohydrate drinks are: Ultra Fuel®, GatorLode®, Exceed High Carbohydrate®

 *** Examples of metabolic optimizer drinks are: Pro Optibol®, Endura Optimizer®, Metababol II® and Muscle Pep®

3 Competition Nutrition

> "The only way to keep your health is to eat what you don't want,
> drink what you don't like, and do what you'd rather not."
> —*Mark Twain*

INTRODUCTION

Haphazard eating habits during the day of competition can exact a heavy toll. At some point, almost all athletes run into problems which better food choices might have prevented: impaired endurance, difficulty concentrating, decreased strength and undue weight loss.

Competition places special demands on your body, and you must be physically prepared to meet those demands. The starting point is sound nutritional knowledge and practice. Yet dedicated competitors, who will sacrifice so much to excel, often ruin their chances with an inefficient and sometimes harmful pre-event diet, inadequate fluid and fuel intake during competition, and sometimes miss the immediate window of opportunity after competition to refuel their muscles.

With some basic knowledge of food and fueling strategies during the competition days, it is usually simple to reverse the situation. If you have ever competed at a disadvantage, read on, because you will learn how to turn competition nutrition into a performance advantage.

PRE-EVENT NUTRITION

Carl was new to the sport of bicycle road racing and, although he had trained hard over the last few months, he continued to "get the bonk, or hit the wall" about halfway through long road races. Mary was competing in a local Tuesday night soccer league. The games started about one hour after she got off work, and she found on numerous occasions that she could not make it through 90 minutes of hard competition without feeling totally fatigued.

Both athletes share a common dilemma. They have not given their muscles the proper food to fuel them through a hard race or game. Their training program and muscles had not failed them — their pre-event diets had. Whether you are an Olympic athlete competing in a marathon or simply training for a high level of fitness, the principles behind fueling-up properly before competition are crucial for optimal performance, as is proper training for competition.

What Happens to Fuel Stores During Competition?

Of the three fuels (carbohydrates, fats and proteins) available to form energy for muscular contraction, only carbohydrates and fats are used to any great extent during exercise. In fact, given an unlimited supply for energy production, the working muscles seem to prefer carbohydrates because its energy contents are easily released and used by the body.

During moderately-hard, prolonged exercise, such as distance running, cycling, cross-country skiing, soccer and basketball, glycogen (stored carbohydrate) and fatty acids (useful form of fat) are both used as fuel sources. During high-intensity exercise such as sprinting, however, glycogen becomes the primary form of fuel for muscular contraction.

Unfortunately, the amount of glycogen stored in the muscles is relatively small compared to what is necessary for long-term exercise. Although the exercising muscles must have carbohydrates, tests performed at the International Center for Aquatic Research at the Olympic Training Center in Colorado Springs show that when carbohydrates are the primary fuel source, muscle and liver glycogen can easily be exhausted in 60 to 90 minutes of hard exercise.

Because the body can run out of carbohydrates, energy must be derived from fat stores in the body. There are abundant supplies of fat even in the thinnest of athletes (about 60,000 to 90,000 calories of fat stored in various parts of our body) — enough fat energy to run 600 to 900 miles. There's one problem: energy from fat stores cannot be supplied quickly to the muscle cells and requires more oxygen to metabolize. Because of this, the glycogen content of the muscles decreases if carbohydrate is not replaced. Fatigue occurs when glycogen in the active muscles used during exercise becomes seriously depleted.

Running Out of Fuel

Remember in Chapter 2, we discussed that a typical 150-pound man stores about 1,800 calories worth of carbohydrate in the muscles, liver and blood. If this individual enters a marathon and maintains a fairly high intensity, he will be burning about 100 calories per mile. While he is burning some fat, he is primarily relying on glycogen for fuel. Those 1,400 calories of glycogen stored in his muscles would run out about 22 miles into the race.

Interestingly, it has been shown that glycogen depletion can also occur during high-intensity exercise that is repeated several times during competition or training. For example, a swimmer who completes several intervals at above his maximal oxygen consumption (highly anaerobic exercise) can also deplete his glycogen stores rapidly.

Carboloading: Endurance Nutrition

Obviously, the primary way our athletes mentioned above can avoid fatigue associated with low glycogen stores is to consume a diet high in carbohydrate prior to competition. The practice of consuming higher carbohydrates before competing is known as "carbohydrate loading" or "glycogen supercompensation."

Carbohydrate loading usually means including an even greater proportion of carbohydrates in your diet. We have been recommending a diet of 60 percent carbohydrate during training. With "carbo loading" you will need to increase your intake to about 70 percent at least two to three days before your event.

Classic Regimen for Carbohydrate Loading

In the 1970's the classical regimen of glycogen loading became very popular. The technique involves depleting carbohydrate stores (glycogen) through intense training for three days and maintaining a low-carbohydrate diet during this time period by eating a diet high in protein and fat. This three-day "depletion" phase is followed by a period of three days of carbohydrate intake of 70 percent. This process allows a trained athlete to increase muscle glycogen stores by 2 to 2.5 times. The results are longer performance times to exhaustion even though glycogen utilization is greater.

However, this method does have its drawbacks. Maintaining training efficiency when carbohydrate stores are low, during the "depletion" phase, is not an easy task. The quality of the workouts suffer, and the risk of injury increases during this three-day period. Many athletes felt that they were not properly prepared if training was dramatically reduced three days before competition. In addition, few athletes want to train to exhaustion 4 to 5 days before competition.

Modified Regimen

Fortunately, Dr. Michael Sherman of The Ohio State University has shown that glycogen supercompensation can be obtained by following a procedure, referred to as the "Modified Regimen" for carbohydrate loading.

Dr. Sherman's recommendations involve the ingestion of about a 50 percent carbohydrate diet for three days, followed by a 70 percent carbohydrate diet for three days during the six days prior to competition. During this six-day period, exercise duration is progressively decreased from 90 minutes on day one, to about 40 minutes on days two and three, to about 20 minutes on days four and five, to a very light day or total rest on day six. This method has been shown to raise glycogen levels comparable to those seen in the more severe "classical" regimen, with fewer side effects. Often, athletes who practice the classical method experience very low levels of energy during the days when very little carbohydrate is consumed due to low blood glucose levels. Figure 3.1 shows how to proceed with the modified regimen for carbohydrate loading.

Days	1	2	3	4	5	6	7
Exercise Duration (minutes)	90	40	40	20	20	rest	Race
Diet (% of calories from carbohydrate)	50%	50%	50%	70%	70%	70%	
OR	4 g carbohydrate/kg body weight/day			At least 10 g carbohydrate/kg body weight/day			

Figure 3.1. The modified regimen for supercompensating muscle glycogen before competition.

The Need for Depletion

Muscle glycogen supercompensation occurs only after your muscles have become depleted. During the depletion phase you train your muscles to become better at using fat as a fuel during exercise, thus, you will use glycogen more sparingly during competition. It also trains your muscles to become better at storing glycogen, so that when you enter the days of high carbohydrate feedings, your muscles become "supercompensated" with glycogen.

That Bloated Feeling

Some athletes have complained of feeling bloated or having heavy legs after a week of high carbohydrates and reduced training. It is a known fact that you store between 3 to 5 grams of water with every gram of carbohydrate. This is what gives one that "heavy" feeling. We suggest that you try carbo loading in training or before a minor competition to see if you experience this feeling, rather than before a major competition. There has been no consistency in the reports of gains in body weight with changes in muscle glycogen levels. But, there may also be an advantage to gaining this "water" weight before competition in the heat. This extra water can be used to help cool you down by providing more water for sweating during high-intensity exercise in the heat.

Events Where It Will Make the Difference

Carbohydrate loading, as we have seen, is a useful tool for helping athletes avoid "hitting the wall." It is unlikely that you will hit the wall in a 10K running race, 1500 yard swim or in an hour game of basketball. However, these athletes should still taper a few days before competition and eat a high-carbohydrate (70 percent) diet during the day or two before the event. To be truly effective your event should be 60 to 90 minutes or greater for carbohydrate loading to be a maximum benefit. Table 3.1 suggests events in which carbohydrate loading will help make a difference.

Table 3.1. Examples of sports suitable for glycogen supercompensation.

Appropriate Activities	Inappropriate Activities
Long-distance swimming	Swimming races
Cross-country skiing	Downhill skiing
Soccer	Weightlifting
Triathlons	Rowing events
Long-distance cycling	Football games
Marathon	Most track & field events
Swim training	

Have You Ever Tried to Eat a 70 Percent Carbohydrate Diet?

It is difficult to eat a diet that is 70 percent carbohydrate. Remember that gram for gram, carbohydrates contain less than half the calories of fat. Once again, you can use high-carbohydrate drinks such as GatorLode®, Ultra Fuel® and Exceed High Carbohydrate® to supplement your carbohydrate intake. These will allow you to consume large amounts of carbohydrate without providing much bulk.

In addition, try to eat a large portion of the 70 percent carbohydrates in complex carbohydrates. Foods such as cereals, pasta, breads, grains and beans will provide you with vitamins, minerals, fiber and protein, as well as carbohydrates. Try to refrain from an abundance of products that contain simple sugars since they tend to be low in vitamins, minerals and fiber. The rest of the diet should contain foods that are good sources of protein and fat.

EATING FOR COMPETITION ────────────

Most athletes are concerned about the timing, type and volume of food to eat before competition. While we will give you some basic suggestions and guidelines to follow, one must not forget that inadequate training or improper daily diet cannot be rectified by your pre-competition meal. Your performance will depend on what you have eaten in the previous days and weeks before the event.

Secondly, the meal before competition needs to be satisfying and psychologically pleasing. You need to enter the event physically, nutritionally and mentally peaked. Consuming foods that you are familiar with and like to eat may give you that needed edge for peak performance.

Fasting Before Competition

Never enter an event with an overnight fast or after long periods of not eating. Although vigorous exercise should be undertaken on an empty stomach, fasting for an extended period of time prior to competition will be counterproductive. Eating several hours before competition replenishes liver glycogen stores to ensure that adequate energy is available. The liver relies on frequent meals to ensure that it stays "tanked-up" with glycogen. If you were to fast for 6 to 10 hours prior to your event (or for that matter a training session), you may experience a premature lowering of blood glucose during exercise. Remember, your liver is a prime source of glucose supply during rest and exercise.

Work conducted by Dr. Edward Coyle, from the University of Texas, has shown that a low-fat, carbohydrate meal containing 75 to 150 grams (300 to 600 calories) of carbohydrates during the final 3 to 4 hours before competition helps to ensure adequate liver and blood glucose stores.

When to Eat and Compete

The timing of your last meal before competition will depend on the intensity and duration of the competition. Begin by experimenting with the timing of your meals. Plan on having your last meal 2 to 4 hours before exercise, and try to move it as close as possible to the start of the event. You want to enter most events with an empty stomach at the time of competition, yet you don't want to feel hungry or weak on the line or starting block.

Additional factors that affect eating and exercise timing are fitness level, exercise intensity and stress. A highly fit individual can perform more intense exercise after eating without placing a great burden on the digestive system. Mild exercise, such as easy cycling and walking, a short while after eating can be tolerated by many athletes. For example, in the Tour de France many athletes can be seen eating on the starting line, since they know the first few hours of the race will be at a moderate pace and they may be racing for up to seven hours. Being nervous about competition will also affect how much and how far before competition you decide to eat.

Table 3.2 gives you some suggestions on what to eat and the timing of meals. For most of us, different start times require different

---

Table 3.2. Pre-race Menus. Here are some suggestions for meals prior to competition for individuals 140 to 170 pounds. Increase or decrease calories slightly according to body weight.

7:00 am Start

Even though this is an early start, you must eat some food before the start. Eat a small amount of high-carbohydrate food (300 to 500 calories) about 1 to 2 hours before the start.

2 to 3 slices of wheat toast and 1 banana
or 1 to 2 cans of a sports nutritional supplement

11:00 am Start

Because of the late morning start, you can eat a regular size breakfast (about 1,000 calories) 3 to 4 hours before the start.

1 cup of oatmeal with fruit
1 cup of skim milk
2 English muffins with jelly
1 blueberry muffin
8 fl oz high-carbohydrate drink

7:00 pm Start

Begin the day with a low-fat breakfast and lunch, and a late afternoon high-carbohydrate snack.

Breakfast (approx. 700-800 calories):

4 pancakes with syrup
1 cup mixed fruit
1 cup skim milk
8 to 12 fl oz of orange juice

Lunch (approx. 800-900 calories):

2 cups spaghetti with tomato sauce
1 slice whole-grain bread
8 fl oz juice
2 pieces fruit

Late Afternoon (approx. 400-500 calories):

1 sports bar
8 to 16 fl oz high-carbohydrate drink

---

meal planning. Just remember that the timing of your pre-event meal really is an individual matter. Although most athletes feel that eating 2 to 4 hours before competition is best, you may find that you need more or less time to digest that last meal.

What to Eat

A major rule to follow before competition is to select foods and drinks that are both physiologically and psychologically pleasing to you, and that your stomach can tolerate well. Best of all, it should be foods that you are accustomed to eating. The day of competition is not the time to try a new exotic breakfast. If you are use to eating pancakes and some juice before your event, do not experiment with a Mexican omelet and fruit if you are from New England and racing in San Antonio. Wait until after the race to experiment with the local cuisine. You may increase your chances of experiencing gastrointestinal distress when experimenting with new foods, especially if you are prone to a nervous stomach.

Here are some simple rules to follow: Once again, high-carbohydrate meals are best, about 70 percent of the meal. Pancakes, waffles, cereals, pasta, bagels, toast, fruit, fruit juices and liquid carbohydrate supplements are all good food choices. During competition, you want to maintain your blood glucose levels and allow for a sustained release of food from your stomach. A combination of simple and complex carbohydrates will allow this to happen.

Carbohydrates can normally be consumed up to one hour before exercise. However, it is wise to experiment with the timing, amount and type of carbohydrate (solid, complex, simple, liquid) in your pre-exercise meal. Ingest 1 to 4 grams of carbohydrate (4 to 16 calories) per kilogram of body weight in the 1 to 4 hour period before competition. If eating one hour before competing, you should eat 1 gram/kilogram; whereas if you decide to eat 4 hours before competition, you should consume 4 grams/kilogram. Experiment with the eating regimen that works best for you.

Avoid meals that are high in protein. Keep the protein content to no more than 10 to 15 percent. Protein foods take longer to digest and absorb. If the pre-event meal is a large steak and eggs breakfast, it will take longer to digest and therefore be in your stomach when the competition starts. In addition, protein foods tend to increase urine output, which can lead to increased dehydration — another good reason to avoid protein before competition or training.

Stay away from diets high in fat, only 15 to 20 percent of the pre-competition diet should be fat. Fried foods, doughnuts, cheeses, foods high in butter and cream cheese, and meats that are high in fat should be avoided. Fat tends to leave the stomach slowly, and some athletes complain of feeling bloated after consuming a high-fat meal.

You do want some protein and fat in your diet; not only do you need these fuels for long-term energy supply, they will help moderate the release of carbohydrates from your stomach. This will help maintain blood glucose levels and ward off hunger pangs in events lasting several hours.

If you are on the road and eating in restaurants, refer to Table 3.2 for our suggestions on your pre-game meal. The principles of satisfying nutritional requirements are no different on the road, but it is often more difficult to carry out the program effectively.

Lastly, if you don't want to be searching for a restroom in the middle of a long race or game, stay away from foods that are high in fiber and fructose. Whole wheat, bran cereals, fresh fruit with skins such as apples, pears and most raw vegetables are high-fiber foods. Some individuals experience gastrointestinal distress and diarrhea when they consume high portions of fructose from juices or fruit before competition or training.

What if I Have to Compete Several Times in One Day

Swimmers, track cyclists and wrestlers are just a few examples of athletes that must compete several times a day during a meet. So, over the hours of a meet, you need to supply energy from carbohydrates to maintain your carbohydrate supply and glycogen stores in your liver. Maintaining your liver glycogen stores will help keep your blood sugar levels at an optimum level. As a result you can prevent feelings of weakness that are caused by blood sugar dips below normal levels.

Scheduling food and drink breaks will help meet your energy needs. If your events are short or intermediate distance and you have approximately three hours between heats or rounds, you may be able to eat a small meal composed primarily of carbohydrates.

Use the same guidelines as described above for the pre-competition meal, but keep the portions smaller. This means eating small amounts of complex and simple carbohydrate meals before your scheduled competition times, so that your stomach is empty during the next round or finals.

Many of the Olympic Team swimmers and cyclists like to experiment with liquid food supplements at this time. Liquid food supplements such as GatorPro®, Nutrament®, Sport Shake® and Exceed Sports Nutritional®, which are complete meals, empty from the stomach quickly and leave little residue that may cause intestinal distress.

Most liquid food products contain between 300 and 500 calories per 8 ounce can, an ideal amount for between sessions. In addition, you may wish to keep sipping carbohydrate beverages during this time.

One might try "energy bars" as a good between-event or pre-race meal. Many of these products are high in carbohydrates and low in fats and proteins. Both liquid food supplements and energy bars can be packed easily in your event bag and are easy to digest. Tables 3.3 and 3.4 give information on both types of food fuels. Make sure to

Table 3.3. Liquid food supplements.

Sports Nutritional Beverage Comparison Chart

Beverage	Calories 8 oz serving	Carbohydrate (grams)	Fat (grams)	Protein (grams)
GatorPro	360	58 (65%)	7 (17%)	16 (18%)
Nutrament	240	34 (57%)	6.5 (25%)	11 (18%)
Sport Shake	310	45 (58%)	10 (29%)	11 (13%)
Exceed	360	54 (60%)	9.5 (24%)	14 (16%)
Go	190	27 (56%)	3 (13%)	15 (31%)
Sustacal	240	33 (55%)	5.5 (21%)	14.5 (24%)

Metabolic Optimizer Beverage Comparison Chart

Beverage	Calories 8 oz serving	Carbohydrate (grams)	Fat (grams)	Protein (grams)
Endura	260	57	<1	11
Metabolol II	260	40	2	20
ProOptibol	266	44	2	18
Muscle Pep	260	45	1	18

High Carbohydrate Beverage Comparison Chart

Beverage	Carbohydrate (type)	Serving Size (ounces)	Carbohydrate (grams/ounce)	Percent Carbohydrate
GatorLode	Maltodextrin & glucose	12	5.9	20
Exceed	Maltodextrin & sucrose	32	7.1	24
Ultra Fuel	Maltodextrin	16	6.25	23

Table 3.4. Sports/Energy Bar Composition Chart

Bar	Size (ozs)	Calories Total	Calories % Carbs	Calories % Protein	Calories % Fat
PowerBar	2.25	225	75	17	8
Exceed	2.9	280	76	17	7
Edgebar	2.5	234	75	17	8
X-Trainer	2.25	220	73	18	9
Tiger Sport	2.3	230	70	19	11
Thunder Bar	2.25	220	74	18	8
Ultra Fuel	4.87	490	82	12	6
Clif Bar	2.4	252	80	8	12
GatorBar	2.25	220	87	5	8
Forza	2.5	231	78	18	4
BTU Stoker	2.6	252	73	16	11
PR Bar	1.6	190	40	30	30
GlycoBar	1.8	180	69	17	4

experiment with both products in training so you are familiar with the taste and how well they settle in your stomach.

If you are one to have a nervous stomach before competition, you may also want to experiment with these liquid food supplements. These products are available in various flavors, and once again it would be wise to experiment before a training session with these products before using them in competition.

Up to the Last Minute

Eating and/or drinking sugar (glucose, sucrose) in the final hours before competition will provide your muscles with an extra dose of carbohydrates for fuel. However, most athletes tend to shun this practice. In the past it was suggested that the consumption of carbohydrates before exercise may elevate blood insulin at the start of exercise which could then lead to a lowering of blood glucose during exercise.

Recently, research has shown that these responses are transient and probably do not affect your performance. Comparison of the new and old studies suggest that individuals differ in susceptibility to a lowering of blood glucose during exercise; the physiological basis for this difference has yet to be determined. Carbohydrates taken in intermittently during the last two hours preceding exercise will ensure that your liver glycogen is topped off and blood glucose levels are high.

At this time, you should be advised that consuming sugar 30 to 60 minutes prior to exercise could harm your performance *if you* are sensitive to a lowering of blood glucose levels. You should test this in training.

You should also consume adequate fluids in the final hours and minutes before competition. Drink about 8 to 12 ounces every 30 minutes during the final hours before competition. Pre-exercise hydration is extremely important. Don't rely on the fluid you consume during the event to help avoid dehydration.

Eat, Drink and Be Faster

In general, the pre-competition meal should be high in carbohydrates and low in fats and proteins. It should also contain adequate amounts of liquid to ensure that you enter the competition well hydrated. After that you need to adjust the timing and types of foods to ensure that they are pleasing and will be adequately emptied from the stomach on the starting line. Most of all your final meal should include foods you know will help your performance, whether it be pancakes, pasta, or a ham or bologna sandwich.

Record your pre-race or pre-game diets in your training diary and see which foods help improve or hinder your performance. Keeping track of the foods eaten, timing of consumption, and how you felt prior to and during the event will be valuable information to your continued success.

The key to success lies in the proper combination of training and nutrition. Take the time to determine that proper combination and don't change much on race or game day.

TOP-FLIGHT COMPETITION NUTRITION ──────────

Susan was tired. She was riding in a 100 mile bicycle ride in 95 degree heat. As she started the last 25 miles of her ride, she wondered, was the ride really worth it? In addition, she had run out of food at the 50-mile mark.

With only one water bottle, high humidity, and several hills left, her speed began to be slower and slower. There was no escape from the heat, humidity and hills.

She was dehydrated, slightly disoriented and not feeling very well. Other experienced cyclists were feeling the same sudden weakness and throbbing in their heads. The high temperatures, heat stress and not having enough fluids was taking its toll on all competitors.

Performance and your health are jeopardized when adequate amounts of fluids and food are not consumed during long-term events, even when the environmental conditions are not so severe. If inadequate replacement fluids and fuels are not consumed during long-term exercise, dehydration, glycogen depletion and low-blood glucose levels can occur. This ultimately leads to reduced endurance, strength and performance.

With the wealth of information available on fluid replacement and eating during events and the expensive advertising about sports drinks and energy bars, it is amazing how many athletes overlook the importance of these practices during endurance training and competition.

Environmental Stress and Dehydration

It is not uncommon for you to lose one to two quarts of fluid via sweating during an hour of training and/or competition. If this fluid is not replaced during exercise, the resulting dehydration will limit your ability to compete and increase your risk of heat injury.

Your body strives to maintain a relatively constant temperature, even during exercise. While some of the heat produced by metabolism is used to maintain body temperature, excessive heat is produced during exercise and you must dissipate this heat to the environment in order to prevent your body temperature from rising to dangerous levels. Add to this increased temperature and/or humidity during competition in the summer months and it becomes even harder for your body to rid itself of heat.

Heat exchange between you and the environment occurs in four ways. While cycling or running into the wind, convective cooling occurs as your body moves through the air. During swimming excessive body heat can be lost by conduction; heat is conducted from your body to the cooler water. Heat can also be lost by radiation, provided that your body temperature is greater than the temperature of your surrounding environment.

However, the most important mechanism for heat loss during exercise under most circumstances occurs with the evaporation of sweat from your skin into the air. Should you fail to ingest enough fluids during long term exercise, the resulting dehydration will reduce your ability to sweat and lead to a progressive rise in your body temperature, predisposing you to premature fatigue and risk of heat illness — just as we saw with Susan earlier.

Sweating is a vital thermoregulatory response at the expense of maintaining your body fluids. Unless you try to keep fluid intake in pace with your sweat loss, sweating will result in dehydration. Fluid losses of as little as two percent of body weight can lead to decreases in performance. For example, if you weigh 150 pounds a weight loss of three pounds of fluid via sweating will have an affect upon performance.

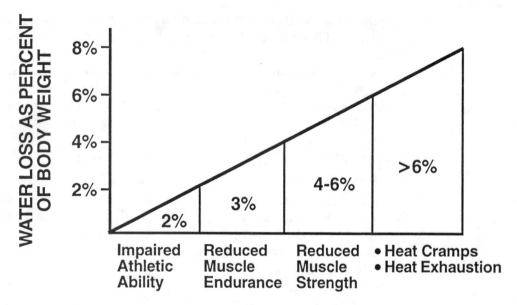

Figure 3.2. Effect of water loss on athletic performance.

When you exercise intensely in hot and humid conditions, your problem worsens because the combination of heat and humidity make it much more difficult for your body to thermoregulate properly. High temperatures and humidity decrease your ability to lose heat by radiation, convection and evaporation. As a result, your body temperature may increase rapidly. Combine the effects of higher environmental heat stress, increased metabolism and dehydration, and exercise becomes a formidable task.

Shrinking Fuel Stores

Marathoners talk of "hitting the wall." Cyclists speak of "bonking." Both groups attribute their fatigue in long events to drained fuel stores. As we have seen, we all have enough fat in our bodies to perform unbelievable endurance events. It's your carbohydrate stores that limit how long you can train or compete.

Remember, the carbohydrate stores of an active 140 to 160 pound man total about 1,800 calories. Of these, 1,400 calories are in the muscles, where they can be used directly; 320 calories are in the liver, and can be released into the bloodstream; and about 80 calories are in the blood, and can travel to anywhere they are needed, including the brain, which can only burn sugar.

Along with replacing fluids, your muscles and brain also need a continuous supply of carbohydrate energy. When you exercise for longer than 60 to 90 minutes, blood glucose levels start to dwindle. After one to three hours of continuous cycling, running or swimming at 65-80 percent of maximum effort, or after repeated bouts of intense sprinting at 85 percent plus of maximum effort, muscle glycogen stores may become depleted. In addition, if only water is being consumed, blood glucose levels may be very low (hypoglycemic) and will result in higher use of muscle glycogen. You may lose your ability to concentrate and react quickly since the brain can only function off of blood glucose.

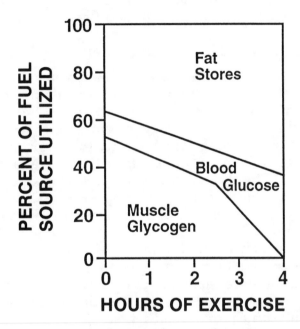

Figure 3.3. Energy sources during prolonged exercise at 70 percent of aerobic capacity. Blood glucose needs to be maintained after 2 to 3 hours of exercise because it becomes the primary source of fuel.

When muscle glycogen levels are low and blood glucose levels have dropped — no matter how fast you may want to go in a race — your body cannot respond, and you have "hit the wall." During exercise, carbohydrates either in liquid or solid form appear to benefit performance by providing an additional source of energy.

Fluid and Energy Replacement During Exercise

You can help maintain your body's supply of carbohydrates by consuming about 25 to 35 grams of carbohydrate every half hour you exercise. Most 8 to 12 ounce servings of sport drinks provide about 15 to 20 grams of carbohydrate, so drinking 8 to 12 ounces every 30 minutes should help you fight off the "bonk."

Drinking plain water, which is fine for events lasting less than 60 minutes, is far better for your body than not drinking at all during competition. However, recent research has shown that your body will absorb more fluid from a sport drink (that contains electrolytes like sodium) than just plain water. So, even during shorter events you may want to consider a sport drink, too, especially if you sweat heavily. Lastly, research has shown that most athletes will consume more fluids that are flavored versus non-flavored beverages.

But What is the Best Energy Drink?

The major goals of fluid supplementation during endurance competition are to provide 1) water and 2) carbohydrate. Water is of the greatest importance, because as we have seen dehydration greater than 2 percent of body weight greatly reduces performance. The purpose of adding carbohydrates to sport drinks is to supplement the limited amount of carbohydrate that's available in your body.

The carbohydrates in sport drinks prolong endurance by providing additional supplemental energy. The carbohydrates are available for fuel within 15 to 20 minutes after you consume them and are almost completely used up during endurance competition. Carbohydrates also help in short-term, high-intensity competition; they allow you to sustain a higher intensity effort than when fats are the primary fuel. Another reason for adding carbohydrates to energy drinks is because in combination with sodium, they enhance water absorption from the intestine into the bloodstream.

Sodium is an essential electrolyte. Its most important functions are to maintain the volume of fluid found outside our cells and to regulate blood volume. Inactive people lose little sodium, but athletes — may lose as much as one gram per hour when they sweat. After exercise, the more rapidly we can replace the water, carbohydrate and sodium we have lost (rehydrate), the more rapidly we can recover.

Rapid absorption of fluid from the small intestine is dependent on sodium. In the presence of sodium, the transport of carbohydrate into the body is dramatically accelerated. This is where sport drinks come into play. Where sodium goes, water quickly follows. To take advantage of this physiological response, sports drinks contain sodium. The sodium found in sport drinks allows athletes to take advantage of this physiological response.

Although some people think of other electrolytes (potassium, chloride, magnesium) as being important during exercise, they play a minor role, except in ultraendurance competition. For most individuals, electrolyte losses other than sodium are low during exercise and will have little negative effect upon performance. However, in ultraendurance events such as the Ironman Triathlon, electrolyte losses may be significant, but most of the time are only seen in athletes who ingest only water during ultraendurance events and not sport drinks. In most sport drinks, the primary reasons for adding sodium is to help replace losses in sweat and to increase the rate that water and carbohydrates get absorbed from your intestine into your bloodstream.

Most energy drinks are between 6 and 10 percent carbohydrate — the percentage that most scientists feel is the proper concentration to optimize fluid absorption and provide carbohydrate to power your muscles and fight off fatigue.

Sport drinks contain either simple or polysaccharides (complex carbohydrates). Simple carbohydrates are sugars such as glucose, fructose and sucrose; polysaccharides are similar to those starches found in bread and pasta, such as glucose polymers or maltodextrin. The better formulated drinks contain both polysaccharides and simple carbohydrates in proper proportions to aid with gastric emptying, usually with a higher concentration of complex carbohydrates as listed by the first ingredient on the label. Higher concentrations of maltodextrins tend to result in less gastrointestinal (GI) distress and stomach ache problems when athletes wish to consume large volumes of sport drinks. However, we should mention that research has shown that there is no difference between drinks containing simple versus complex carbohydrates as far as being absorbed from the intestine into the blood stream.

Stay away from drinks that contain a large amount of fructose (usually listed first on the ingredient list). This sugar can slow down gastric absorption and can cause GI problems in some people. If fructose is added as a second ingredient for sweetness and energy, however, its concentration is less and doesn't seem to have any adverse effects.

Lastly, if you can get your hands on a cool fluid during competition, by all means drink it. Cool fluids empty faster from your stomach than warm fluids. They also taste better, which will cause you to drink more. And, by now you know, the more sport drinks you consume, the better your performance.

Super-Hydration Drinks

The first major breakthrough in fluid replacement performance drinks in several years, may be on the horizon. Not since the introduction of carbohydrate polymers has there been much exciting information to report to you on "fluid replacement" drinks. But new research

Table 3.5. Fluid Replacement Comparison Chart

Beverage	Carbohydrate Type	Carbohydrate Concentration per 8 oz	Sodium (mg)	Potassium (mg)
PowerAde	High fructose corn syrup & maltodextrin	8	73	33
Gatorade	Sucrose & glucose	6	110	25
AllSport	High fructose corn syrup	8-9	55	55
10-K	Sucrose, glucose, fructose	6.3	54	25
Cytomax	Fructose corn syrup & sucrose	7-11	10	150
Breakthrough	Maltodextrin, fructose	8.5	60	45
Everlast	Sucrose, fructose	6	100	20
Exceed	Glucose polymers, fructose	7	50	
Hydra Fuel	Glucose polymers, fructose, glucose	7	25	
Hydra Charge	Maltodextrin, fructose	8		trace
Coca-Cola	High fructose corn syrup	11	9.2	trace
Orange juice	Fructose, sucrose	11-15	2.7	510
SportaLYTE	Maltodextrin, fructose, glucose	7.5	100	60

indicates that athletes can get a head start on hydrating (similar to carbohydrate loading) before competition or training.

Maximizing hydration is important, since dehydration carries with it two big negatives for athletes: (1) Each 2 percent drop in body weight can significantly lower one's ability to produce power (and thus speed). For example, athletes can easily lose 2 percent of their body weight during one hour of cycling in the heat or two hours of swim or wrestling training. (2) Excessive dehydration can also increase the risk of heat exhaustion and even heat stroke.

Cycling speed declines primarily because dehydration reduces the water portion of the blood (plasma) and subsequently decreases blood volume. Less blood is sent to the muscles to provide fuel and oxygen and to the skin to help with cooling. With the quantity of blood reduced, heart rate and body temperature climb, and competing at race pace is more difficult. Although drinking fluids during competition helps prevent dehydration, emptying of fluids from the stomach often cannot keep pace with high sweat rates.

For the last ten years scientists have been investigating ways to prevent or at least limit the negative effects of dehydration. Now, Dr. Paul Montner and co-workers at the University of New Mexico Veterans Hospital have found a safe and natural chemical that can do the job. The substance is glycerol, which is found naturally in many foods and is added to many processed foods. Their research has shown that when glycerol is ingested prior to exercise, blood volume remains high, heart rate remains lower, and performance improves.

In their original study reported in *Medicine and Science in Sports and Exercise* (Vol. 24(5): S157, 1992) , 11 trained cyclists drank a glycerol-water drink before one ride and an artificially flavored (plain water) drink before another. During both rides the cyclists rode at a moderately high intensity, under laboratory conditions, for as long as possible. When water was ingested, the cyclists were only able to ride 77 minutes; but when glycerol was ingested along with water, they were able to ride for 94 minutes. During the glycerol trial, blood volume was preserved and body temperature and heart rates were lower compared to the water trial.

This preliminary study showed that glycerol when assimilated into the blood acts like a "sponge" which absorbs the water into the blood and holds it there. More water in the blood allowed for increased blood volume and more moderate heart rates and for more blood to be sent to the skin for cooling and to the muscles to help with energy production.

Recently it was reported by Dr. E. W. Askew in an article detailing the use of glycerol in *Olympic Coach* (Vol. 3(3):12, 1993) that soon we may be seeing sport drinks on the market to help athletes achieve a state of optimal hydration. While glycerol is a safe food additive, athletes should use a source of glycerol which is suitable for human consumption. Glycerol, also called glycerine or glycerin, can be found in many pharmacies. Currently, Dr. Askew is recommending that the dose of glycerol taken in with fluid should not exceed one gram per kilogram (2.2 pounds) of body weight every six hours.

A loading program may include taking glycerol with adequate amounts of water or a sports drink about 90 minutes before competition or training. You should also continue to hydrate every 30 minutes leading up to the start of the race. This will give the glycerol a chance to move out of the stomach and into the bloodstream before you begin riding. During a very long race (four or more hours) you may consider taking in some additional glycerol along with fluids at about the three hour mark.

Some athletes testing relatively higher doses of glycerol have reported symptoms of nausea, bloating and lightheadedness after consuming glycerol. As with any drink or food, glycerol may be tolerated differently by each individual. You should try hydrating with glycerol in practice several times before trying it on race day. None of the subjects in the New Mexico study reported problems. It may be assumed that they were using the right amount of glycerol, and if they consumed larger amounts they may have experienced these symptoms.

While glycerol may not make a camel out of you, it can help optimize hydration when ingested with fluids. Thanks to this recent research, you may see energy drinks containing glycerol soon, but you must remember to also consume drinks that contain between 6 and 10 percent carbohydrate before and during competition to ensure that blood glucose levels are maintained — and that your muscles are recharged with glycogen. Athletes need to maintain blood volume and blood glucose levels during exercise. Glycerol and carbohydrate containing sport drinks can help prevent fluid losses and the lowering of blood glucose which can impair judgment, aerobic efficiency, reaction time and performance.

Fast Track Snacking

Some individuals do not like drinking excessive amounts of fluids during endurance exercise. Some nutritionists have suggested that exercise induced nausea can be accentuated by having liquids sloshing around in your stomach for long periods of time. Eating solid foods which contain carbohydrates and small amounts of proteins and fats may help settle the stomach when large volumes of fluid are being ingested.

In addition, many people crave something solid to eat after being on the road for many miles. If you are competing in events lasting over several hours, it might also be wise to consume some solid food during the event. This food will not only supply carbohydrates, but will give you a sense of having solid food in your stomach (satiety) and not leave you with that empty feeling in your stomach. Several products are available to eat during exercise that are good tasting and will not upset your stomach. Many of the energy/sport bars on the market contain similar amounts of carbohydrate, but are better for you than a standard high-fat candy bar or cookie. Research has shown that during endurance exercise as much as 10 percent of your energy may come from protein stores, so some protein in a bar will aid with energy and also help during recovery when your muscles are hungry for amino acids. Make sure to consume some fluid along with these bars.

Remember these points when eating energy bars during training or competition:

1. Drink several ounces of fluid with the energy bar, especially during exercise when you need the fluids in addition to the energy from the bar.

2. Stay away from bars that are high in protein and fat. The primary fuel that you use during exercise is carbohydrates, which should be first on the ingredient label.

3. Eat before you are hungry. Waiting until you are hungry will mean that your blood glucose and muscle glycogen stores may be too low for peak performance.

4. During cold weather racing or training, some energy bars will need to be kept close to your body to prevent freezing.

5. If riding a bicycle, drink at the end of the pace line if on a bike, while the pace is slow, and when the road is free of hazards, and not while climbing or descending at fast speeds.

Check the label of the bar to ensure that they are high in carbohydrate and low in fat and protein (see Table 3.4). Select bars that are over 80 percent carbohydrate and less than 10 percent fat. Remember there are 4 calories per gram of carbohydrate, 4 calories in each gram of protein and 9 calories per gram of fat. A bar than contains 11 grams of fat and 5 grams of protein in a bar containing 225 calories is 44 percent fat calories, about 50 percent carbohydrate calories, and 9 percent protein calories.

Recently, a new type of bar has appeared on the market which contains 40 percent of its calories from carbohydrate and 30 percent from both fat and protein. The developer claims the product will improve your ability to burn fat during a workout or race. The higher concentration of protein is said to stimulate the release of the hormone glucagon, which, in turn, releases more fatty acids into the blood and spare blood glucose. These higher fat bars are also suppose to spare more muscle glycogen by allowing you to burn more fat during exercise, thereby, improving endurance. While there is plenty of antidotal evidence by athletes to show they work during long-term exercise, many in the scientific community do not see any validity to their claims.

Other research is currently being conducted at several universities on the use of medium chain triglycerides, better know as MCTs. MCTs are lipids that act like a carbohydrate and tend to be burned for fuel rather than being stored as a fat. MCTs will be discussed in greater detail in Chapter 6.

For the current time the vast majority of research collected over the last 30 years has shown that without carbohydrates during exercise, fatigue will set in quicker, and you will "bonk" or "hit the wall" before the finish. By consuming carbohydrates you may still tire, but you may be able to push the pace longer and harder.

Carbohydrate-rich foods, like fresh fruits as well as breads and cereals and energy bars along with athletic drinks, are important tools in the nutritional arsenal of any athlete. The secret is to try different forms of carbohydrates (solid vs. liquid, bar vs. food) and find the one that works best for you. In some cases it may be a combination of solid and liquid, like a banana and sport drink, during a one- or two-hour workout. Whichever one works best for you is the one to use in training and competition — taste and palatability are your biggest concerns. Keep the carbohydrate content high and fat content low, and your energy levels will remain high.

Quick Energy

Move over energy bars — a new high energy concentrated form of carbohydrate gel is being marketed to performance athletes. You can discover new endurance by carrying this convenient, efficient energy source. Each package of premeasured carbohydrate (80 to 100 calories) can be consumed during exercise.

"They deliver quick energy for sustained levels of performance. When taken with water or an energy/sports drink they will maintain blood sugar levels and maximize endurance and performance," says Deborah Kelly, Vice President of New Business, for Gatorade, who is now distributing ReLode®, their introduction to this product category. Several other carbohydrate gel products on the market are Pocket Rocket®, GU® and Squeezy®.

This product is perfect for that last 10 miles in a long race or tour when you need that quick burst of energy. "We have been experimenting with Pocket Rocket with our riders in long road stages, and find them to deliver quick energy to help sustain high levels of performance," points out Chris Carmichael, Coaching Director for the U. S. Cycling Team. But remember, when using these products it is important to stay well hydrated. It is important to still use an energy drink or water during long road races. These products contain a high carbohydrate concentration and if not properly used they can decrease gastric emptying and increase the risk of dehydration and gastrointestinal distress.

This type of product can also be used immediately after exercise to help with recovery. Ingesting 1 to 2 packets of a carbohydrate gel, along with at least 10 ounces of water or energy drink with each packet, can enhance glycogen resynthesis rate. Carbohydrate gels are not designed to totally replace energy drinks or bars during exercise, but to give you that extra shot of pure carbohydrate during endurance competition.

As more and more carbohydrate gels and other forms of sport nutritionals come onto the market, we recommend experimenting with these products in training as with any new food or drink product. Take

Table 3.6. Carbohydrate Gel Comparison Chart

Packet	Size (ozs)	Calories	Grams Carbs
Pocket Rocket	1.25	100	25
ReLode	0.75	80	20
Squeezy	1.0	100	25

the opportunity to taste several of the products and experience what it is like to use the gel packet during exercise or a metabolic optimizer during prolonged exercise.

Nutritional Sense

Obviously, there are a number of alternative ways to meet your nutritional needs during long duration exercise. If you are going to experiment with sport drinks, bars, gels and different fuel replacement patterns, make sure you do so in training first. Don't wait until race day to experiment with foods and fluids. Do not become a victim of stomach cramps, GI problems or dehydration because you did not practice eating and drinking in training. With some judicious trial and error, you will discover the feeding pattern that works best for you.

Nutrition and fluid replacement play a critical role in successful training and event participation. You have trained hard, purchased the proper equipment and have toned your skills. Developing and designing the proper nutrition and hydration strategies may be all you need to perform closer to your potential. Optimal fluid replacement and efficient intake of carbohydrates during training and racing is an essential component in achieving top physical performance.

POST-EVENT NUTRITION ─────────────

The race is over, you pack up your equipment and drink about 10 to 12 ounces of water. After collecting your prize, you jump into your car and drive the three hours home before you sit down to a meal.

The next day you're tired the whole day and, even after a good warm-up, you still feel sluggish during your workout. For many years people have told you that you just went too hard in the race and may not have had enough training or yardage in order to recover from such a hard race. We now know better.

Your muscles and liver have not completely refilled themselves with glycogen, which is the sugar that's stored in the liver and muscles, and is of primary importance in sustaining power output during exercise. Research has shown that workouts or races that last over 60 to 90 minutes can put severe demands upon your body's glycogen stores. If the workout was long and hard enough, your muscles may even "bonk" during the event.

In addition to endurance exercise, high-intensity exercise can deplete your glycogen stores rapidly. As little as 10 intervals lasting 90 to 120 seconds can severely deplete your carbohydrate stores. A hard session of basketball, training on the track or alpine skiing will reduce your stores to empty in no time. So if you train or compete in sports like swimming, soccer or basketball, your muscles will most likely be depleted of glycogen.

Recovery: Crucial to Future Performance

Generally, athletes and coaches have not considered post-event nutrition as important as pre-event eating or nutrition during the event. Following the completion of hard training or competition, it may take up to 24 hours to resynthesize muscle glycogen provided ample carbohydrate is consumed.

As we have seen there may be times when you will train or compete several times a day, so it is important to rebuild muscle and liver glycogen stores as quickly as possible. Because stores of glycogen are essential for maximum performance, you may need to regenerate these energy stores as rapidly as possible. Research has repeatedly shown that when no carbohydrate is consumed after exercise, very little glycogen synthesis occurs over the next 24 hours.

Timing

In recent years, John Ivy, Ph.D. has conducted a series of studies at the University of Texas that has shown that properly timed carbohydrate feedings can optimize the restoration of muscle glycogen stores. In one study, Dr. Ivy and co-workers, gave cyclists either a placebo or 2 grams of glucose per kilogram (2.2 pounds) of body weight immediately after and 2 hours after cycling, or 2 grams of glucose per kilogram only 2 hours after cycling. Muscle biopsies, taken immediately after the ride and 4 hours post-exercise, showed that glycogen synthesis was the highest when the cyclists were fed immediately post exercise.

The group that consumed carbohydrate immediately after exercise showed a 300 percent increase in the glycogen resynthesis above the resting group during the recovery period. The group that consumed carbohydrate 2 hours after exercise showed a 46 percent slower rate of glycogen synthesis, compared to the group ingesting carbohydrate immediately after exercise.

The moral of the story is to eat carbohydrate as soon as possible after exercise. This is especially true if you are working out or competing twice or more in one day. If you do one workout in the morning and one in the evening, time is of the essence if you hope to ingest enough carbohydrate to restore glycogen stores.

Replacing Fluid and Fuel

Noting the results of several studies, Michael Sherman, Ph.D., in a presentation at the 1992 Olympic Marathon Trials, suggested that consuming carbohydrate every 15 minutes after exercise produced a slightly higher rate of muscle glycogen resynthesis than consuming carbohydrate at 1 or 2 hour intervals. He suspects that the significant increase in muscle glycogen results, by keeping insulin and blood glucose elevated, by eating more often — an important factor in optimal storage of glycogen.

Based upon this particular information and your particular situation you should consume at least 0.75 gram carbohydrate per kilogram of body weight every hour (Method A), or 1.5 gram of carbohydrate per kilogram, immediately after exercise and every 2 hours thereafter (Method B), or consume 0.4 gram carbohydrate per kilogram of body weight every 15 minutes after exercise (Method C).

The following table provides a schedule for implementing these three strategies for individuals of various weights who consume a liquid high carbohydrate at least 20 percent carbohydrate (e.g., 20 grams carbohydrate/100 ml [3.6 ounces]). Examples of such products are Gatorlode® (20%), Exceed High Carbohydrate® (24%) and Ultra Fuel® (23%).

Table 3.7. Volumes of liquid carbohydrate to consume during the hours after exercise or competition to replenish muscle glycogen.

Weight		Method A		Method B		Method C	
(lb)	(kg)	(ml)	(oz)	(ml)	(oz)	(ml)	(oz)
100	46	175	6	345	12	92	3
150	68	255	9	510	18	136	5
200	90	340	12	675	24	180	7

The liquid carbohydrate source is 20% carbohydrate (e.g., 20 grams carbohydrate/100 ml (3.6 oz). Method A= volume consumed immediately after exercise and every hour thereafter; Method B= volume consumed immediately after exercise and every 2 hours thereafter; Method C= volume consumed immediately after exercise and every 15 minutes thereafter.

Why Liquid Supplements

Immediately after strenuous exercise your appetite may be suppressed. Therefore, eating solid foods right away may not be appealing. However, most of us will be thirsty and need fluids. By drinking a sports drink or high carbohydrate beverage we can rehydrate and refuel at the same time. As we have seen, ingesting carbohydrate at the end of training or competition can stimulate glycogen replacement, thereby shortening recovery time and allow you to practice or compete the next day with more available energy.

Endurance Builders

Metabolic optimizers are nutritionally complete powders. Their combinations of protein, fat, carbohydrate, vitamins, minerals, and sometimes herbs, are designed to not only replenish depleted glycogen (carbohydrate) stores, but to aid in recovery of muscle tissue of essential amino acids and other nutrients after hard exercise. Their nutritional breakdown reflects a balanced approach toward nutrition for endurance athletes: approximately 65-70% carbohydrate, 20-30% protein and less than 10% fat. These products are sold under the names of Muscle Pep® (Sports Pep), ProOptibol® (Next Nutrition), Metabolol II® (Champion Nutrition) and Physique® (Shaklee).

Research conducted by Dr. John Ivy, from the University of Texas, has shown that protein in combination with carbohydrates in a recovery drink, turns on the metabolic switch of increased insulin secretion (hormone which allows carbohydrate and protein to enter cells) which stimulates greater uptake of both carbohydrate and protein into the muscle [*Journal of Applied Physiology*, 72(5): 1854-1859, 1992]. Insulin is your body's principal anabolic "on-off" switch. It moves into the blood stream and sets your muscle rebuilding wheels in motion.

Dr. Ivy discovered that the right balance of protein with carbohydrate produced a greater secretion of insulin into the blood than did either carbohydrate or protein alone. Metabolic optimizers provide a blend of protein and carbohydrate blend to help rebuild your muscles. As with standard high carbohydrate drinks, you should consume 1.0 to 3.0 grams of a metabolic optimizer powder per kilogram (2.2 pounds) of body weight within 30 minutes of finishing a hard exercise session. For example, a 150-pound cyclist would consume between 68 and 204 grams of a metabolic optimizer after a long, hard training ride or race.

While being promoted primarily as pre- and post-exercise nutritional supplements, optimizers may have other advantages in endurance cycling. "Cyclists are also experimenting with metabolic optimizers during long road races (120 miles plus) where it has been shown that not only is carbohydrate an important fuel, but that cyclists also begin to use amino acids (protein) for fuel after carbohydrate stores become depleted," states Steve Hegg, professional cyclist with the L.A. Sheriffs/Chevrolet cycling team.

"Carbohydrate and possibly protein from such products can spare the breakdown of muscle tissue by supplying protein in the later stages of exercise," points out Chris Carmichael, Coaching Director for the U. S. Cycling Team. Many of the newer optimizer powder drinks are easy to mix just with water, which makes them as convenient to use as standard powdered energy drinks at the race site (see metabolic optimizer section of Table 3.3).

Chronic Dehydration

Checking your morning body weight on a daily basis while in hard training can determine if you are chronically dehydrated. If you are down several pounds from the day before, you are chronically dehydrated. The weight loss is in fluid not fat as some athletes believe. You should be within a pound of your previous day's weight; if not, you will enter that day's event or training dehydrated. This will surely affect your performance and lead to increased chances of overheating and early fatigue.

Make sure to have several glasses of energy drinks, juices, skim milk or water with all your meals. Drink fluids throughout the whole day, not just before the workout or race. Chronic dehydration is as harmful to your performance as chronic glycogen depletion.

Double Workouts

Dr. Carl Foster, physiologist for the U. S. Speed Skating Team, had the team consume a high-carbohydrate beverage immediately after the end of hard training sessions. In the next workout session, he found that performance improved, and they did not feel as if they had worked as hard. Improved performance has also been shown in soccer players who drank a high-carbohydrate drink between successive games. The athletes who drank the high-carb drink were able to play at a higher intensity and cover more ground in the second match, compared with the players who only had water and no carbohydrate intake.

But I Like Solid Food

If solid food is more to your liking in the hours after exercise, consider this example for consuming carbohydrates immediately after, and 2 and 4 hours post-exercise. For instance, a 150-pound individual could drink 16 to 30 ounces of a high carbohydrate beverage immediately after exercise; followed by a meal at 2 hours that includes several cups of pasta or rice, vegetables, bread and some protein foods; followed at 4 hours (maybe an evening snack) of an apple, bagel and carbo drink.

Type of Carbohydrates

The type of carbohydrate that you consume can also affect the rate of glycogen synthesis. Recent nutritional research has indicated that foods with a "high-glycemic index" actually increase the amount of resynthesis of glycogen faster than foods classified as "low-glycemic index" foods. High glycemic foods are defined as foods that raise one's blood glucose levels rapidly after exercise. For example, glucose and bread are high-glycemic index foods and resynthesize your muscle glycogen stores twice as rapidly as fructose or beans which are low-glycemic foods. In order to insure rapid and full rebuilding of glycogen stores, consume foods that have a high-glycemic rating. Avoid those foods that will delay glycogen resynthesis.

Daily Carbohydrate Needs

In Chapter 2 we saw that the need to eat every day affects your recovery and ability to train or compete at maximum effort and effectiveness. Hard training, including long sessions or intervals at high-intensity, will deplete your reserves of muscle and liver glycogen. It will take a full 24 hours to restore your glycogen stores after a tough workout, but you must consume from 8 to 10 grams of carbohydrate per kilogram of your body weight in this time period.

So after your initial dose or two of carbohydrate, you'll want to ensure that you get in your desired 8 to 10 grams of carbo's per kilogram of body weight. For example, a 155-pound athlete, weighs 70 kilograms, and needs to consume between 560 and 700 grams of carbohydrate a day (8 x 70 = 560 grams). Table 2.1 in Chapter 2 shows foods high in carbohydrate that should be eaten with every meal to ensure that you get in 8 to 10 grams of carbohydrate per kilogram of body weight or a minimum of 60 percent of your daily diet.

Should you take in your carbohydrate in several small meals or in a few large meals? Studies show that it doesn't matter whether you eat two or three large meals or seven small meals during a 24-hour period after a strenuous workout; the rate of glycogen resynthesis is about the same, as long as the total carbohydrate intake is equivalent. If you have two hard and long workouts on one day, you will have to eat more

Table 3.8. Glycemic Indices of Some Foods

High Glycemic Index	Low Glycemic Index
glucose	milk
white bread	ice cream
potato, baked	pear
carrots, cooked	fructose
honey	plum
banana	yogurt
white rice	peach
rice cakes	grapefruit
	carrots, raw
Medium Glycemic Index	peanuts
raisins	dried peas
macaroni	dried beans
sucrose	kidney beans
orange	
orange juice	
yams	
sweet potato	
oatmeal	
grapes	
apple	
spaghetti	
peas	

than 8 to 10 grams per kilogram of body weight per day in order to be ready for your next day's activities.

RECOVERY: CRUCIAL FOR FUTURE PERFORMANCE

Once competition or strenuous training has ended for the day, nutritional management once again becomes important for future performance. Since you must recover from the stress of competition and return to normal as soon as possible, your body's energy and fluid reserves must be restored rapidly.

So the moral of the story is the same. If you want to train consistently and compete at your best, eat high-carbohydrate diets. About 60 to 65 percent of your total caloric intake should be carbohydrate. Stress carbohydrates in the pre- and post-exercise meals. Fluids and carbohydrates should be ingested as soon as possible after the end of exhaustive exercise. Avoiding chronic glycogen depletion and dehydration is crucial for your next day's racing or training.

4 Basic Nutrition for Good Health and Performance

"Tell me what you eat, and I will tell you what you are."
—*Anthelme Brillat-Savarin*

INTRODUCTION

Nutrients are life-sustaining substances obtained from food. They work together to supply athletes with energy to build muscle, perform and maintain health. Protein, carbohydrate, fat, vitamins, minerals and water are the six major classes of nutrients. (Table 4.1 lists nutrient categories and their functions.)

Only three of the six classes of nutrients provide energy. They are protein, fat, and carbohydrate. Energy for the body is supplied primarily by carbohydrate and fat. Only a small amount of protein is used for body fuel. Vitamins, minerals and water do not supply energy. Their role in the diet is to help break down the energy found in food. Carbohydrate and protein provide about half the energy that fat provides. (Table 4.2 lists the energy found in protein, carbohydrates and fat.)

WHAT IS PROTEIN?

Protein is necessary to build and maintain all body cells. Since cells are constantly being replaced, protein is needed daily. Protein is used to:

- maintain and repair muscles and other body tissues
- make hemoglobin, which carries oxygen to the exercising muscle
- form antibodies in the blood that fight off infection and disease
- produce enzymes and hormones that regulate the body processes
- supply energy, when carbohydrates and fats are not sufficiently consumed

Protein is made up of amino acids. When protein foods are eaten, these amino acids are absorbed and used to form muscles, hemoglobin, enzymes, and hormones. Contrary to popular belief, protein is not a

55

Table 4.1. The six classes of nutrients and their major functions.

NUTRIENT	FUNCTION
PROTEIN	• Build and repair body tissue • Major component of enzymes, hormones, and antibodies
CARBOHYDRATE	• Provide a major source of fuel to the body • Provide dietary fiber
FAT	• Chief storage form of energy in the body
VITAMINS	• Help promote and regulate various chemical reactions and bodily processes • Do not yield energy themselves but participate in releasing energy from food
MINERALS	• Enable enzymes to function • A component of hormones • A part of bone and nerve impulses
WATER	• Enables chemical reactions to occur • About 60% of the body is composed of water • Essential for life as we can not store it nor conserve it

Table 4.2. Energy yielding nutrients and their caloric value.

CARBOHYDRATE	4 calories per gram
FAT	9 calories per gram
PROTEIN	4 calories per gram

primary source of energy, except when athletes are not consuming enough calories or carbohydrates. If a swimmer's diet is not balanced, or if total daily caloric intake is insufficient, protein will be broken down and used as an energy source instead of being used for its intended job of tissue building. Excess amino acids that are not used to form tissues, enzymes or hormones are converted and stored as fat, and the excess nitrogen found in these amino acids is sent to the liver and converted into urea and then sloughed off in the urine.

Historically, athletes felt they needed a high-protein diet to have the "strength of a bull." Although protein provides the basic building blocks for muscles, consuming more protein than what the body can use will just give an athlete the most expensive urine in town. Concerns regarding excessive protein intake also include a monetary perspective; some of these protein supplements cost in excess of $50.00 per day.

Protein Requirements

The Recommended Dietary Allowances for healthy people in the

United States lists protein requirements on a per-weight basis. The suggested range of protein requirements for athletes is 0.8-2.0 grams of protein per kilogram of body weight. Training and competitions may promote a loss of muscle protein via reduced protein synthesis and increased protein breakdown. Thus, a 17-year-old male swimmer who weighs 145 pounds needs from 53-132 grams of protein per day. To determine your own protein requirement use the equation found in Table 4.3.

Table 4.3. Equation for calculating protein requirements.

To determine your protein requirement:

Take your weight in pounds _____ and divide by 2.2 _____ (that is your weight in kilograms).

Take your weight in kilograms _____ and multiply by 1.5 _____ (that is your protein requirement per day).

For example: 154 lbs. ÷ 2.2 = 70 kilograms of body weight
70 kilograms x 1.5 = 105 grams of protein per day.

To determine the amount of protein foods you need to eat, use the following as a guide:
- 8 grams of protein are in 1 cup of milk, yogurt, or 1 ounce of cheese
- 7 grams of protein per ounce of meat (beef, chicken, fish)
- 3 grams of protein per serving of bread or grains (1 slice of bread, ½ cup of rice, ½ cup of pasta)

The typical American diet supplies about 100 grams of protein per day, 70 percent from animal sources which contain all the essential amino acids, for a total protein intake of about 1.4 grams per kilogram of body weight. So you can see, most consumers as well as athletes meet or exceed their protein requirements.

Usually, athletes consume more protein when their caloric intake increases as a result of training. For example, a 70 kg athlete who gradually increases his caloric intake from 2,500 calories to 5,000 calories during training would increase his protein intake from 75 to 150 grams per day if 12 percent of his calories came from protein.

Athletes can obtain 1.2 to 2 grams of protein per kg when their diet provides 12 to 15 percent of calories as protein. This amount of protein is consistent with the dietary recommendations for athletes. The growing athlete has a greater need for protein relative to body weight than does a mature athlete. A diet supplying 15 percent of the calories from protein should meet the needs of most growing athletes.

Problems With Too Much Protein

Athletes who eat enough calories and have reasonably balanced diets don't need protein supplements because their diet already provides enough protein. There is no evidence that protein supplements are effective for promoting endurance or strength. When more protein is consumed than the body can use, the excess protein is either burned as energy or stored as fat. (Table 4.4 lists potential problems with high protein diets.) Consuming large amounts of protein at the expense of carbohydrates can lead to chronic fatigue in athletes due to low-muscle glycogen stores. In addition, consuming a high-protein, high-fat diet after strenuous exercise will cause slow or incomplete replacement of muscle glycogen.

Table 4.4. Potential problems with high protein diets.

- Excess protein is converted to fat
- Protein foods are generally more expensive
- Foods high in protein may contain more fat
- Increased protein in the diet may inhibit the replacement of muscle glycogen
- Takes longer to digest if used as a pre-game meal
- Requires more water to eliminate the extra nitrogen, which may lead to dehydration

Consuming too much protein, whether through food or supplements, increases the body's water requirement and may contribute to dehydration. The metabolism of protein requires more body water than carbohydrates and even fat, and, therefore, when dietary protein increases, increased water is recommended to minimize dehydration. If athletes are consuming large amounts of protein, they should be made aware of the importance of increasing fluids in their diets.

There is also a potential problem with excessive protein intake in female athletes. Women who consume large amounts of dietary protein have higher calcium excretions. Women who consume large amounts of protein in combination with low-calcium diets may be at risk for osteoporosis.

There is a group of athletes who may not be getting enough protein on a daily basis. Usually they are athletes who participate in lean profile sports such as gymnastics, diving, figure skating, judo or any other sport that has restricted weight classifications. These athletes are usually on some type of low-calorie, weight-restricted diet. They eat so few calories that they don't consume enough protein or carbohydrate, fat or vitamins and minerals. When athletes severely restrict their caloric intake, protein requirements actually increase. Protein requirements increase because it is being used as a fuel source to satisfy their energy needs instead of carbohydrate or fats. If the athlete stays on a low-calorie diet longer than 3 days, muscle mass will be lost rather than fat stores (see Chapter 7 for more details on proper methods for weight loss).

Amino Acid Supplementation

Health food stores and popular magazine articles advertise a wide variety of protein and amino acid supplements, and people take them for various unfounded reasons. Athletes take them to build muscle, dieters take them to spare their bodies protein while losing weight, and women take them to strengthen their fingernails. As is the case with many other magic solutions to health and fitness, protein and amino acid supplementations do not work and can be harmful.

Proponents of amino acid supplementation claim that their products are more rapidly digested and absorbed than protein found in food. They also claim that certain amino acids increase muscle mass and decrease body fat. The body is designed to handle whole proteins, like those found in food, best. When proteins are predigested in a laboratory and served up as mixtures of amino acids, the cells in the intestines cannot accommodate them all at once; so fewer amino acids are digested and absorbed. In contrast, about 95-99 percent of the protein from animal sources and about 90 percent of the protein from vegetable sources are digested and absorbed by the body — giving the advantage to food protein not amino acid supplements. (Table 4.5 shows examples of protein rich foods for meeting protein requirements.)

Table 4.5. Protein amounts found in common foods.

Food	Portion Size	Protein (grams)
Milk (skim, 2%, whole)	1 cup	8
Yogurt (nonfat, low-fat)	1 cup	8
Cheese (any variety)	1 ounce	8
Lean hamburger patty	3 ounces	26
Egg/egg white	1	7
Lean steak	3 ounces	21
Chicken breast	3.5 ounces	30
Taco	1	11
Pizza	2 slices	32
Tuna	3 ounces	24
Peanut butter	1 tablespoon	4
Whole wheat bread	1 slice	3
Pasta	1 cup	6

Amino Acid Supplementation Concerns

Substituting amino acid supplements for food may cause deficiencies of other nutrients found in protein-rich foods such as iron, niacin, and thiamine. Another concern is that the use of single or unbalanced amino acid supplements may interfere with the absorption of certain essential amino acids, leading to a protein deficiency. When athletes consume too much of a single amino acid, it creates an imbalance and may bind with other essential amino acids leading to a negative nitrogen balance and loss of protein from the body.

High-protein diets are also usually high in fat. Consuming a high-protein, high-fat diet after strenuous exercise will cause slowing or incomplete replacement of muscle glycogen and, therefore, impair performance.

As mentioned earlier, excess amino acid and protein supplementation which cannot be incorporated into new proteins are either burned as energy or converted into fat. When amino acids are burned for energy or converted to fat, excess urea production results, which may increase the risk of dehydration. The kidneys need more water and have to work harder to eliminate the extra nitrogen load imposed by the excess protein.

Ingestion of single amino acids like ornithine can cause mild to severe stomach cramping and diarrhea. Other amino acids alter brain neurotransmitter activity and some, such as methionine, are very toxic.

There is no scientific evidence that supplementation with specific amino acids will increase muscle mass or decrease body fat. Also, there may be as yet unidentified long-term risks associated with amino acid supplementation. It makes absolutely no sense to consume a product which has not been proven safe or effective — particularly when that product is promoted by individuals who stand to gain financially.

FAT

In a typical American diet about 35-40 percent of calories consumed are in the form of fat—an amount that has been linked to an increased risk of obesity and heart disease. Although fat is an energy source (9 kcal/gram of fat), athletes are advised to limit fat in their diets, as even the leanest of athletes have more body fat than is needed during a workout. A high-fat diet also decreases the intake of carbohydrate. It is widely accepted that no more than 30 percent of the total daily calories should come from fat. Keep in mind some key points about fat:

- Fat takes longer to digest than protein and carbohydrates and, therefore, may still be in the stomach at the start of exercise or during exercise. For this reason athletes are advised to consume minimum amounts of fat before and during exercise.
- Consuming a high-fat diet compromises carbohydrate intake which may lead to chronic fatigue.
- In order to burn fat as a fuel source the body must have sufficient carbohydrate levels to use fat effectively as energy.

Fat Budget

A personal fat budget is based on body weight and caloric expenditure. Use Table 4.6 to figure your personal fat budget. Fat budgets are based on weight maintenance, and if an athlete wants to lose weight, a fat budget at or below the current diet should be chosen.

The goal of the fat budget is not to eat more fat than has been budgeted. Using Table 4.6 you can figure how much fat you should be consuming. For example, a 19-year-old female swimmer who is concerned about how much fat she can eat, should limit her fat intake to between 70 and 90 grams of fat per day. If she desires to lose weight, she needs to eat fewer grams of fat.

Becoming familiar with high-fat foods and not exceeding one's fat budget will help you eat more carbohydrates and less fat, so you will have the energy to train and become a better athlete. Some athletes cut out an entire food group, thinking the foods are all high in fat, but there are low-fat foods in every food group. Table 4.6 shows the grams of fat in each of the five food groups. Use them to select the lower fat foods and stay within your fat budget.

Types Of Fat

Fats are made up a glycerol backbone with three fatty acids (Figure 4.1). Fatty acids may differ from one another in two ways: in chain

```
G — Fatty acid
L
Y
C — Fatty acid
E
R
O
L — Fatty acid
```

Figure 4.1. Triglyceride

Table 4.6. Your fat budget.

The best way to keep your fat consumption under control is to "budget" it. Everyone can have a fat budget . . . which is the amount of fat you can reasonably eat each day and meet current dietary guidelines that 30 percent of calories or less come from fat. For example, if you are eating 3000 calories per day, multiple 3,000 by 30 percent to determine the maximum number of calories that should be coming from fat in one day. (3000 x .30 = 900 calories from fat). One gram of fat equals 9 calories, divide the calories from fat by 9 to see how many grams of fat you should be eating per day (900 ÷ 9 = 100 grams of fat per day). Use this table to find your total daily fat.

Daily Caloric Intake	Calories from fat per day	Maximum gram fat per day
1200	360	40
1400	420	47
1500	450	50
1600	480	53
1800	540	60
2000	600	67
2200	660	73
2400	720	80
2600	720	87
2800	840	93
3000	900	100
3200	960	107
3400	1020	113
3600	1080	120
3800	1140	127
4000	1200	133
4200	1260	140
4400	1320	147
4600	1380	153
4800	1440	160
5000	1500	167

By simply adding up fat grams in foods you consume using the food lists below or food labels (see Appendix C), you can easily evaluate your fat intake . . . without ever dealing with percentages and calculators.

Watch your portions
Understand that "what" you eat is only half of the equation. "How much" you eat is just as important. For example, one tablespoon of dressing on your salad is "budgeted" at 5 grams of fat. Two tablespoons "cost" double that. Learning to eat smaller portions of fat is a valuable trick.

If you want to lose weight
Fat budgeting can easily be used as a method to help you cut down on unwanted fat calories. If you would like to lose weight, select a fat budget one or two levels below your current calorie intake. Make sure you are still at a calorie level that allows you to train and compete. With a slight decrease in fat and a calorie level that still allows you to train, you will lose weight.

Table 4.6. (*Continued*)

FAT CONTENT OF SELECTED FOODS

MILK GROUP	FAT (grams)*
American cheese (1 oz)	10
Cheddar cheese (1 oz)	10
Parmesan cheese, grated (1 oz)	10
Ice cream, 16% fat (1 cup)	10
Chocolate milk, 2% (1 cup)	5
Mozzarella cheese, (1 oz)	5
2% milk (1 cup)	5
Instant pudding (½ cup)	5
2% Cottage cheese (½ cup)	3
Ice milk, soft serve (½ cup)	3
1% milk (1 cup)	3
Fruit flavored yogurt (1 cup)	3
Frozen yogurt, plain (1 cup)	1
Skim milk (1 cup)	0
Plain, nonfat yogurt (1 cup)	0

*Fat grams have been rounded for easier addition

MEAT GROUP	
Polish sausage (3 oz)	25
Ground beef, broiled (3 oz)	20
Dry roasted peanuts (¼ cup)	20
Quiche, (¼ pie)	20
Beef hot dog (1)	15
Peanut butter (2 TSP)	15
Roast beef, lean and fat (3 oz)	15
Bacon (3 slices)	10
Bologna, beef (1 slice)	10
Fried chicken, batter dipped (3 oz)	10
Fried shrimp, batter dipped (3 oz)	10
Sirloin steak, broiled (3 oz)	10
Canned tuna in oil (3 oz)	7
Salmon, cooked (3 oz)	5
Canadian bacon (2 slices)	5
Hard cooked egg (1)	5
Ham, 5% fat (3 oz)	5
Roast beef, lean only (3 oz)	5
Turkey (3 oz)	5
Roasted chicken, without skin (3 oz)	3
Water packed canned tuna (3 oz)	3
Flounder/sole, baked (3 oz)	1
Refried beans, canned (½ cup)	1
Boiled shrimp (3 oz)	1
Cooked pinto beans (½ cup)	0

FRUIT GROUP	
Avocado, pureed (½ cup)	20
Apple, orange or peach (1)	0

Table 4.6. (*Continued*)

FRUIT GROUP (*continued*)	FAT (grams)
Strawberries (½ cup)	0
Applesauce (½ cup)	0
Orange juice (½ cup)	0

VEGETABLE GROUP	
French fried potatoes (10)	10
Hash browned potatoes (½ cup)	10
Oven-heated french fried potatoes (10)	5
Coleslaw (½ cup)	3
Winter squash, baked (½ cup)	1
All green vegetables (½ cup)	0
Baked potato (1 large)	0
Fresh tomato (1)	0
Tossed salad without dressing (½ cup)	0
Cooked corn (½ cup)	0

GRAIN GROUP	
Homemade waffle (7″ waffle)	10
Stuffing, from mix (½ cup)	10
Boston Chicken's cornbread (1)	8
French toast (2 slices)	5
Snack crackers (4)	5
Plain croissant (½ roll)	5
Granola (1 oz)	5
Bran muffin (1 small)	5
Boston Chicken's rice pilaf (5 oz)	5
Biscuit from mix (1)	3
Pancake (4″ pancake)	3
Flour tortilla (8″ tortilla)	3
Wheat thin crackers (8 crackers)	3
Dinner rolls, brown and serve (1)	2
Triscuit cracker (3)	2
Bagel (½)	1
Oyster crackers (10 crackers)	1
Whole wheat bread (1 slice)	1
Hamburger or hot dog bun (1)	1
Graham cracker (2)	1
English muffin (½ muffin)	1
Oatmeal (½ cup)	1
Corn tortilla (6″ tortilla)	1
Macaroni (½ cup)	0
Spaghetti (½ cup)	0
Corn flakes (½ cup)	0
Rice, wild or white (½ cup)	0

Table 4.6. (*Continued*)

COMBINATION FOODS/FAST FOODS	FAT (grams)
Burger King's Double Whopper w/Cheese	62
Taco Bell's Taco Salad (1)	55
Burger King's Croissant Egg, Ham & Cheese	41
Subway Cold Cut Combo (12 inch)	40
Boston Chicken's Chunky Chicken Salad	38
Taco Bell's Mexican Pizza (1)	38
Hardee's Bacon Cheeseburger	36
Burger King's Whopper (1)	35
Boston Chicken's Chicken Pot Pie (1)	35
Hardee's Frisco Grilled Chicken Sand (1)	34
Taco Bell's Nachos BellGrande (1)	34
Shoney's All American Burger (1)	33
McDonald's Big Mac (1)	30
McDonald's Quarter Pounder with Cheese	30
Pizza Hut's Supreme Personal Pizza	30
Subway Seafood and Crab Sub (6 inch)	29
Subway BMT (6 inch)	28
Arby's Beef and Cheddar (1)	27
Shoney's Country Fried Steak (1)	27
Taco Bell's Big Beef Burito Supreme (1)	25
Homemade Chicken Pot Pie (¼ of 9″)	25
Wendy's Broccoli and Cheese Potato (1)	25
Boston Chicken's Tortillini Salad (5.6 oz)	25
Dairy Queen Double Hamburger (1)	25
Boston Chicken's Creamed Spinach (6.4 oz)	24
Taco Bell's Chicken Burrito Supreme (1)	23
McDonald's Large French Fries (1)	22
Homemade Macaroni and Cheese (1 cup)	20
Pillsbury Frozen French Bread Pizza (1 pc)	20
McDonald's Chicken McNuggets (6 pc)	18
McDonald's McLean Deluxe w/Cheese (1)	16
Arby's Roast Beef Sandwich (1)	15
Peanut Butter and Jelly Sandwich (1)	15
Wendy's Single Hamburger, Plain (1)	15
Taco Bell's Taco Supreme (1)	15
Taco Bell's Soft Taco Supreme (1)	15
Van de Kamps Frozen Beef Enchiladas (1)	15
McDonald's Cheeseburger (1)	13
McDonald's McLean Deluxe, Plain (1)	12
Taco Bell's Bean Burrito (1)	12
Taco Bell's Taco (1)	11
Boston Chicken's Mashed Potatoes w/Gravy	10
Taco Bell's Steak Soft Taco (1)	9
McDonald's Hamburger (1)	9
Chick-Fil-A Chicken Deluxe w/Bun	9
Arby's Roast Turkey Deluxe (1)	6

Table 4.6. (*Continued*)

CAKES/PIES/COOKIES/SNACK FOODS/SWEETS	
T.J. Cinnamon's Cinn Roll (1)	34
Dairy Queen Buster Bar (1)	29
Pecan Pie (⅛ of 9″ pie)	25
Au Bon Pain Carrot Muffin	23
Au Bon Pain Current Scone	23
Dairy Queen Heath Blizzard (1 small)	23
Cheesecake (¹⁄₁₂ of cake)	20
Haagen Dazs Chocolate Ice Cream (4 oz)	17
Doughnut, Yeast Glazed (1)	15
Apple Pie (⅛ of 9″ pie)	15
Dairy Queen Dilly Bar (1)	13
Wendy's Frosty (med)	13
Chocolate Candy Bar, Plain (1 oz)	10
Cream Cheese (1 oz)	10
Mayonnaise (1 TBSP)	10
Potato Chips (10 Chips)	10
Dairy Queen Van. Cone (large)	7
Butter (1 TSP)	5
Chocolate Chip Cookies (2 small)	5
Salad Dressing, Italian (1 TBSP)	5
Coffee Whitener, Nondairy (1 TBSP)	3
Sour Cream (1 TBSP)	3
Pretzels (1 oz)	1
Angel Food Cake (¹⁄₁₂ of cake)	0
Popcorn, Air Popped, Unbuttered (1 cup)	0
McDonald's Soft Serve Cone (1)	0

(Adapted from Healthy Dividends: A Guide To Balancing Your Fat Budget. Western Dairy Council, 1992)

length and in degree of saturation. Chain length affects how the fat mixes with water. The shorter the chain length the more soluble in water. Saturation refers to the chemical structure — specifically, to the number of hydrogens the fatty acid chain is holding. If every available bond from the carbons is holding a hydrogen, we say the chain is saturated. If the bonds from the carbons have a few empty spots, we say the chain is unsaturated. If there is one point of unsaturation, then it is a monounsaturated fat. If there are two or more points of unsaturation, then it is a polyunsaturated fat.

Saturated Fats

Saturated fat is solid at room temperature and is derived mainly from animal food. Saturated fat also raises blood cholesterol: the more saturated fat consumed, usually the higher the blood cholesterol. While saturated fat is usually derived from animal products, there are some animal products that have lower amounts of saturated fat. Table 4.7 lists the amounts of saturated fat found in some animal products.

Unsaturated Fats

Unsaturated fat is liquid at room temperature and is mainly found in plant foods. These types of fat along with a low-fat diet tend to lower blood levels of cholesterol. There are two exceptions to the rule. Two plant oils, that are liquid at room temperature, tend to raise blood cholesterol. They are **coconut and palm oil** and are known as tropical oils. Athletes need to watch for these two oils when reading labels to find heart-healthy foods.

What about vegetable oils that are solid at room temperature . . . like margarine? Should they be classified as saturated or unsaturated? Well, it depends. In order to get a liquid oil solid at room temperature, a process known as hydrogenation has to take place. Basically, hydro-

Table 4.7. Fatty acid content of some fats.

Fats with large amounts of saturated fat (in percentages):			
	Saturated	**Monounsaturated**	**Polyunsaturated**	**Other Lipid**
Coconut Oil	87	6	2	5
Palm Kernel Oil	81	11	1	1
Butter	62	29	4	5
Fat in Whole Milk	62	29	4	5
Lard	41	47	11	1
Fat in Beef	38	44	3	15
Fat in Chicken	28	35	21	16
Fat in Pork	34	45	12	9

Fats with large amounts of monounsaturated fatty acids (in percentages):			
	Saturated	**Monounsaturated**	**Polyunsaturated**	**Other Lipid**
Margarine (tub)	18	39	39	4
Olive Oil	14	74	8	4
Canola Oil	6	62	22	10
Peanut Oil	18	49	33	0

Fats with large amounts of polyunsaturated fatty acids (in percentages):			
	Saturated	**Monounsaturated**	**Polyunsaturated**	**Other Lipid**
Corn Oil	13	24	59	4
Soybean Oil	15	24	54	7
Safflower Oil	11	13	77	0

Note: All fats, whether they contain mainly saturated, monounsaturated or polyunsaturated fatty acids, provide the same number of calories: 9 calories per gram.

genation is simply adding hydrogens to the carbon chain so that every carbon atom is filled with hydrogens. Adding hydrogens to the chain will allow the vegetable oil to become solid at room temperature, however, it also gives the fat the same characteristics of a saturated fat in that it will raise blood cholesterol. In order to choose a heart-healthy margarine, athletes must read the label. If the ingredient lists hydrogenated or partially hydrogenated fat first, then this margarine is **not** heart healthy and will raise cholesterol. On the other hand, if the ingredient lists liquid vegetable oil first and then hydrogenated or partially hydrogenated second or third, this margarine is mostly unsaturated and will be better for your heart. Manufacturers can control the extent of hydrogenation; they do not have to automatically convert all unsaturated fatty acids to saturated fatty acids.

Cis- and Trans- Fatty Acids. Recently, there has been some controversy over hydrogenated fats. When an unsaturated fat is hydrogenated, the configuration around the double bond changes and, therefore, affects it function. The terms **cis-** and **trans-** describe the locations of the hydrogens next to the carbon where the double bond was. As Figure 4.2 illustrates, a **cis-** fatty acid has its hydrogens on the same side, whereas a **trans-** fatty acid has them on opposite sides of the double bond. These arrangements affect the configuration of the fatty acid and in turn affects their functions. The **cis-** configuration is typical of the fatty acids in natural foods, but during hydrogenation, some hydrogen atoms shift around some of the double bonds, changing them to **trans-** bonds. **Trans-** fatty acids are more stable, but

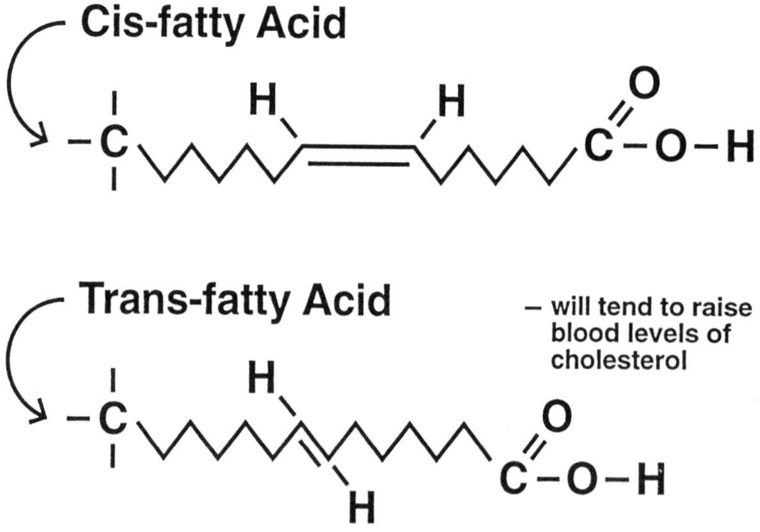

Figure 4.2. Configurations of Cis- and Trans- fatty acids.

their safety is being questioned. Studies have shown that diets rich in **trans-** fatty acids raise low-density lipoproteins (LDL; the bad cholesterol) and lowers high-density lipoproteins (HDL; the good cholesterol) at least to the same extent as saturated fatty acids do. As with trade-offs the choice of which products to use, and in what quantities, is up to the athletes. Given the advice to limit fat consumption, combined with the possible adverse health effects of processed fats, it seems desirable to take advantage of all opportunities to select foods and design meals that are low in fat.

Lowering Fat In The Diet

Athletes need to recognize that there are many sources of hidden fat in the diet. Fat is present, but sometimes invisible. For example, hidden fats exist in dairy products, granola bars, french fries, avocados, chips, nuts, and many processed foods. The other sources of fat are more clearly visible, such as margarine, butter, mayonnaise, salad dressing, oil, and sour cream. Athletes must learn how to lower their consumption of fat, so that they may be able to perform better, as well as lower their chances of heart disease and other lifestyle diseases associated with high-fat intakes. To help lower the fat in your diet, try these simple substitutes found in Table 4.8.

Table 4.8. Fat substitutions.

INSTEAD OF:	TRY:
• Whole milk	Skim milk
• Cheddar, jack or Swiss cheese	Part-skim mozzarella string or low-fat cottage cheese that contains less than 5 grams of fat per ounce
• Ice cream	Ice milk or low-fat/nonfat frozen yogurt
• Butter or margarine	Jam, yogurt, light sour cream, blender whipped cottage cheese
• Bacon	Canadian bacon or bacon bits
• Ground beef	Extra lean ground beef or ground turkey
• Fried chicken	Baked chicken without the skin
• Doughnuts, pastries, breads	Bagels, whole-grain homemade breads, muffins, and quick bread
• Apple pie	Baked or raw apple
• Chocolate candy or bars	Jelly beans, hard candy, licorice
• Cookies, cakes, brownies	Vanilla wafers, ginger snaps, graham crackers, fig bars

CARBOHYDRATES

Athletes receive most of the energy for exercise from ingesting carbohydrate-rich foods. Foods such as breads, cereals, pasta, fruits, vegetables, and dried beans and peas are excellent sources of carbohydrates. Adequate amounts of carbohydrate are essential for athletic performance. Carbohydrates are stored in the liver and muscles as glycogen, and their principle functions are to:

- provide primary energy source for the working muscles
- provide primary energy source to the brain and central nervous system
- help burn body fat more efficiently

Simple Carbohydrates

There are two classifications of carbohydrates: simple and complex. Simple carbohydrates include monosaccharides, which are single or one-sugar units. Disaccharides are two monosaccharides or two-sugar units linked together. Glucose, fructose and galactose are the simple sugars, whereas, sucrose and lactose are two common disaccharides. Sugars in any form — honey, raw sugar, syrup, candy, jelly, or table sugar (sucrose) — have very little nutrients and are all converted to glucose before the body can use it as a fuel. The muscles and brain require blood glucose for energy. As a matter of fact, the only fuel that the brain can use is glucose. When athletes limit the consumption of carbohydrates or skip breakfast, blood glucose levels drop and the brain is poorly supplied with its essential fuel. Consuming adequate amounts of carbohydrates in meals and snacks will increase blood glucose and supply the muscles and brain with its essential fuel. A poorly fueled brain limits muscular function and mental activities such as concentration and mental drive that it takes to perform at one's best.

Complex Carbohydrates

Whereas simple carbohydrates contain glucose, fructose and galactose in single and pairs, complex carbohydrates contain mostly glucose units strung together as polysaccharides. Three classes of complex carbohydrates are important in nutrition: starch, fiber, and glycogen.

Starch

Plants store sugars in the form of starch. For example, corn on the cob, which is sweet when it is young, becomes starchy as it gets older. The sugar is converted to starch. Fruits tend to convert starches to sugars as they ripen. For example, a green banana with some yellow is mostly starch and contains very little sugar, whereas a brown ripened banana is mostly sugar and contains very little starch. Potatoes, rice, and bread are other starches that we eat. These starches are digested into glucose and either burned for energy or stored in the form of glycogen. Starches offer an advantage over simple carbohydrates in the fact that they are more nutrient dense. Meaning they have the same capabilities to fuel exercise, but starches and complex carbohydrates have more vitamins, minerals, and fiber than do simple carbohydrates.

Fiber

Once commonly called "roughage," fiber has attracted much attention in recent years as its role in disease prevention has come to light. Fibers are the structural parts of plants. Most are complex carbohydrates, but they do not include starch. Studies of populations suggest that fiber-rich diets protect against heart disease, colon cancer, and diabetes. The protective health effects of fiber are found not in one magic food but in a high-fiber diet which includes insoluble fibers like whole grains, fruits and vegetables, as well as soluble fibers like oat bran, barley, and legumes (dried beans and peas).

Fibers can be classified according to their solubility in water. The effects of fibers on the body do not neatly divide along the lines of solubility, but some generalizations can be made. In general, soluble fibers occur in higher concentrations in fruits, oats, barley, and legumes. They tend to delay the stomach's emptying time, making you feel full longer, and tend to lower blood cholesterol. In one study about 2 ounces of oat bran was added to a low-fat diet and the subjects' blood cholesterol dropped 5 percent. The subjects actually lowered their risk for heart disease by 10 percent, because for every 1 percent drop in blood cholesterol you reduce your risk of heart disease by 2 percent. By consuming more beans, oat bran, oatmeal, rice, barley, and fruits not only do you have the health benefits of these soluble fibers, but they are also rich in complex carbohydrates and protein, which will help fuel training and competition.

Insoluble fibers are generally found in higher concentrations in vegetables, wheat, and cereals. They relieve constipation and have been found to lower the risk of colon cancer. Insoluble fibers increase fecal weight, absorb water, and make the stool easier to pass. This type of fiber may prevent colon cancer by diluting, binding and rapidly removing potential cancer-causing agents from the colon.

While athletes should be consuming more fiber-rich foods in their diets, consuming them in a pre-race meal may be detrimental to performance, especially if the fiber causes you to make several "pit stops" along the race course. High-fiber foods speed up transit time in the gastrointestinal tract and soften the stool for passage. While this is good for overall health, it may not be good on a race day when the athlete is already nervous and having diarrhea. The recommendation is to keep fiber-rich foods to a minimum in the pre-event meal and consume them post-exercise for the health benefit.

Glycogen

Glycogen, the storage form of carbohydrates found in the muscles and liver, consists of many glucose molecules linked together in highly branched chains. This arrangement permits rapid breakdown. During exercise a hormonal message is sent to the muscles and liver that says "release energy." When this message arrives at the liver or muscle cell, enzymes respond by attacking all the branches of glycogen simultaneously, making a surge of glucose available for energy.

Muscle Glycogen. Depleted muscle glycogen causes athletes to "hit the wall," while depleted liver glycogen causes them to "bonk or crash." During endurance exercise like a marathon, muscle glycogen stores become progressively lower. When they drop to critically low levels, high-intensity exercise cannot be maintained. In practical terms, you are exhausted and must either stop exercising or drastically reduce the pace. Glycogen depletion may also be a gradual process, occurring over repeated days of heavy training, where muscle glycogen breakdown exceeds its replacement. When this happens, the glycogen stores drop lower with each successive day, and you have difficulty maintaining the same training intensity. Figure 4.3 illustrates the glycogen level in the muscles of collegiate swimmers who swam for two consecutive days. Day 1 consisted of two workouts each consisting of two hours. After the second workout, they had ten hours rest. Day 2, the swimmers worked out for two hours in one practice session. After just two days of high-intensity workouts, these swimmers used most of the glycogen in their muscles and did not regain glycogen levels between workouts. Only after rest and consumption of carbohydrates did the swimmers regain muscle glycogen levels.

Liver Glycogen. When the muscles run out of glycogen, they will begin to take up some of the blood glucose, placing a drain on the liver glycogen stores. The longer the exercise session, the greater the utilization of blood glucose by the muscles for energy. When liver glycogen is depleted, blood glucose drops, and you may experience symptoms of

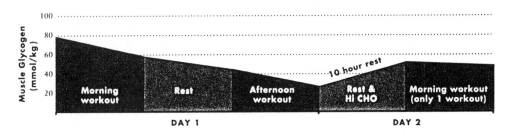

(ICAR Research Annual, 1991-1992)

Figure 4.3. Glycogen depletion in collegiate swimmers after repeated workouts.

hypoglycemia such as dizziness, nausea, light-headedness, and confusion (Figure 4.4). Most athletes note local muscular fatigue and have to reduce their exercise intensity.

The risk of chronic glycogen depletion can be prevented by consuming a high-carbohydrate diet, ingesting a carbohydrate containing sport drink during exercise, and incorporating periodic rest days into the training schedule. To ensure a carbohydrate-rich diet, you should be consuming about 450-550 grams of carbohydrate per day or 4-5 grams of carbohydrate per pound of body weight to restore carbohy-

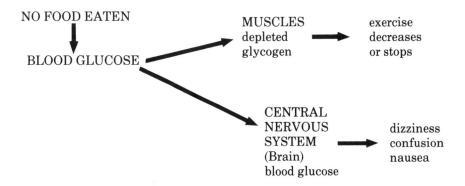

Figure 4.4. Endurance exercise and glycogen depletion.

drate levels and maintain optimal performance. Table 4.9 lists examples and gram weight of high-carbohydrate foods. If you don't want to count grams of carbohydrate daily but want more of a general guide to consuming more carbohydrate-rich foods, Figure 4.5 gives the recommended number of servings from the Food Guide Pyramid. Using these two tools for diet planning, you can provide both the muscles and liver with optimal levels of glycogen for health and performance.

VITAMINS AND MINERALS

Vitamins and minerals are necessary for the growth of all body tissues. They are also essential for the release of energy in the body. While each vitamin and mineral has an important role in maintaining normal cell functions, only small amounts of each vitamin or mineral is needed.

Vitamin and mineral deficiencies can impair physical performance. However, there is no evidence that taking more vitamins or minerals than the body can use will improve performance. In fact, large doses of some vitamins and minerals can be harmful.

Vitamin and Mineral Supplementation

Many athletes take a low-dose multi-vitamin and mineral supplement to give them "peace of mind" that they are getting the proper amount of nutrients needed. In low dosages, these supplements pose little or no risk. There may be some cases where specific vitamin and mineral supplementation is advised. Athletes who are eating low-calorie diets to lose body fat, growing athletes, female athletes, and those who travel regularly may need a vitamin and mineral supplement. However, they should seek the advice of a physician or other qualified health professional before consuming a supplement. (For more on vitamins and minerals see Chapter 5.)

DIET PLANNING

As an athlete, you need about 40 nutrients or so for top performance. How can you select from the tens of thousands of foods available to create a diet that supports health and performance? Generally, by eating a wide variety of foods from the Food Guide Pyramid, athletes should get all of the nutrients they need. No single food or food group supplies all the nutrients an athlete needs. So it is important that athletes choose a wide variety of foods from each group. If they

Table 4.9. Foods listed by groups with carbohydrate content.

High-Carbohydrate Foods

Food Group	Serving	Calo-ries	Carbo-hydrate (Grams)	Food Group	Serving	Calo-ries	Carbo-hydrate (Grams)
Milk							
Low-fat milk (2%)	1 cup/8 oz.	121	12	Frozen yogurt	1 cup	220	34
Skim milk	1 cup	86	12	(low-fat)			
Chocolate milk	1 cup	208	26	Fruit-flavored	1 cup	225	43
Pudding (any flavor)	½ cup	161	30	yogurt (low-fat)			
Meat							
Meat loaf	3 oz.	230	13				
Fruit							
Apple	1 medium	81	21	Grapes	1 cup	58	16
Apple juice	1 cup	111	28	Grape juice	1 cup	96	23
Applesauce	1 cup	194	52	Orange	1 medium	65	16
Banana	1 medium	105	27	Orange juice	1 cup	112	26
Cantelope	1 cup	57	13	Pear	1 medium	98	25
Cherries (raw)	10	49	11	Pineapple	1 cup	77	19
Cranberry juice	1 cup	147	37	Prunes (dried)	10	201	53
Dates (dried)	10	228	61	Raisins	⅔ cup	300	79
Fruit cocktail	½ cup	56	15	Raspberries	1 cup	61	14
(in own juice)				Strawberries	1 cup	45	11
Fruit roll-ups	1 roll	50	12	Watermelon	1 cup	50	12
Vegetable							
Blackeye peas	½ cup	99	78	Pinto beans	1 cup	235	44
Carrots	½ cup	31	7	Potato	1 large	139	32
Corn	½ cup	88	21	Refried beans	1 cup	270	47
Garbonzo beans	1 cup	269	45	Sweet potato	1 large	118	28
Lima beans	1 cup	217	39	Three-bean salad	½ cup	90	20
Navy beans	1 cup	259	48	Water chestnuts	½ cup	66	15
Peas (green)	½ cup	63	12	White beans	1 cup	249	45
Grain							
Bagel	1	163	31	Graham crackers	2 squares	63	11
Biscuit	1	103	13	Saltines	5 crackers	60	10
White bread	1 slice	61	12	Triscuit crackers	3 crackers	60	10
Whole wheat bread	1 slice	61	11	Pancake	1	61	9
Breadsticks	2 sticks	77	15	Waffles	1	130	17
Cornbread	1 square	178	28	Rice	1 cup	206	50
Cereal (ready-to-eat)	1 cup	110	24	Rice (brown)	1 cup	232	50
Cream of Wheat	¾ cup	96	20	Hamburger bun	1	119	21
Malt-O-Meal	¾ cup	92	19	Hotdog bun	1	119	21
Flavored oatmeal	1 packet	110	25	Noodles (spaghetti)	1 cup	159	34
(instant)				Flour tortilla	1	95	17
Supplements							
GatorLode®	11.6 oz.	280	70	GatorPro®	11 oz.	360	59

Source: *The Swimmer's Diet: Eating for Peak Performance*, Gatorade, 1992.

eat at least the minimum recommended number of servings from each group daily, athletes can be reasonably assured that they are getting the nutrients they need for optimal performance. Figure 4.5 lists the minimum recommended number of servings needed by athletes at different times in the season. By following this guide athletes can be nutritionally ready for their competition.

What counts as a serving?

Milk Group:
1 cup of milk or yogurt
1½-2 ounces of cheese

Meat, Poultry, Fish, Dry Beans, and Nuts Group:
2-3 ounces of cooked lean meat, poultry or fish
½ cup cooked dry beans
1 egg
2 tablespoons peanut butter

Vegetable Group:
1 cup raw leafy vegetables
½ cup other vegetables, cooked or chopped raw
¾ cup vegetable juice

Fruit Group:
1 medium apple, banana, orange
½ cup chopped, cooked or canned fruit
¾ cup fruit juice

Bread, Cereal, Rice, and Pasta Group:
1 slice of bread
1 ounce of dry cereal
½ cup cooked cereal, pasta, or rice

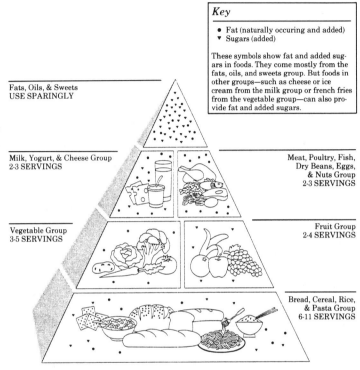

Looking at the Pieces of the Pyramid
The Food Guide Pyramid emphasizes foods from the five major food groups shown in the three lower sections of the Pyramid. Each of these food groups provides some, but not all, of the nutrients you need. Foods in one group can't replace those in another. No one of these major food groups is more important than another—for good health, you need them all.

Servings needed for active individuals.

OFF-SEASON TRAINING DIET 2800 calories		IN-SEASON TRAINING DIET 3300 calories	
Milk	4 or more servings	Milk	5 or more servings
Meat	3 or more servings	Meat	4 or more servings
Vegetable	6 or more servings	Vegetable	8 or more servings
Fruit	4 or more servings	Fruit	6 or more servings
Grain	16 or more servings	Grain	18 or more servings

Figure 4.5. Using the food guide pyramid for wise food choices.

5 Vitamins and Minerals: Team Players

> "Sweat cleanses from the inside. It comes from places a shower will never reach."
> —*George Sheehan*

INTRODUCTION

Because there is confusion in the minds of some athletes over what makes up a nutritionally balanced diet and the fact that most active individuals don't understand the RDA's (Recommended Dietary Allowances), many athletes turn to vitamin and mineral supplementation as nutritional insurance.

The question that arises is should most active people be taking a supplement? Generally no. The athlete who takes a simple one-a-day type of vitamin or mineral supplement that does not exceed the nutrient levels of the RDA is probably not doing any harm. However, recent recommendations from vitamin and mineral researchers are that athletes who take a multiple type of vitamin should do so every three days to reduce the risk of over-supplementation. The concern is for the athlete who has a whole cabinet full of supplements. These individuals take a handful of supplements for breakfast, several tablespoons of nutritional yeast and assorted pills containing trace minerals, powdered protein and herbs throughout the rest of the day. These athletes assume supplements are better than a balanced diet. Takers of self-prescribed supplements need a warning about the risk of overdosing.

VITAMINS

Vitamins are potent organic molecules needed in very small amounts. They cannot be manufactured by the body, and therefore we need to consume them on a daily basis. The amount we need each day totals less than one eighth of a teaspoon, yet without them health, physical performance, and mental function would be severely impaired and death may follow.

Their main function is regulating and facilitating the millions of chemical reactions that take place in the body. They are very rarely destroyed and are able to carry on their function repeatedly.

Vitamins are divided into two major categories, those that are fat-soluble and found in the fatty portions of food and body tissues, and those that are water-soluble and found in the bodily fluids. Vitamins A, D, E and K are classified as the fat-soluble vitamins, while the eight B vitamins and vitamin C are considered water-soluble.

The body can store excess amounts of the fat-soluble vitamins for future use. For this reason, foods rich in these nutrients do not have to be consumed every day. The water-soluble vitamins are far more readily excreted from the body, and daily intakes of these vitamins are needed to maintain tissue levels.

Vitamins are organic compounds necessary in small amounts in the diet. They do not provide the body with energy in and of themselves, however, they do play a role in breaking down and releasing the energy found in food. There are 13 or more of them, and if any one is missing for a period of time then a deficiency disease becomes apparent. The following is a rundown of the 13 major vitamins, how the body uses them, and what foods contain them.

Vitamin A

Vitamin A is a fat-soluble vitamin meaning that it is stored in the fatty tissue like the liver. Most everyone is familiar with its role in preventing night blindness, but it also plays a major role in cell growth and maintaining healthy tissues. A vitamin A deficiency can cause dry rough skin that may become more susceptible to infections.

Research with animals have suggested that excess vitamin A may cause birth defects. The amount needed to cause this harm is not known. There are lethal amounts of active vitamin A. An extremely high dose has been known to cause death. Vitamin A is found in two forms: carotene, the nonactive form which is converted in the body to the active form; and vitamin A itself, formed from carotene and certain food sources such as liver, eggs, and milk. Carotene is found in orange and green vegetables such as carrots, pumpkin, squash, and spinach. It is nontoxic, however, if you overdose on carrots, your skin and the whites of your eyes can turn a yellow-orange color. This is called hypercarotenosis and is not harmful, just a sign of too much carotene.

Vitamin B_1 — Thiamin

This is a water-soluble vitamin and part of the B complex. Thiamin is required for the release of energy from food and for normal digestion, growth, lactation and function of the nervous system.

A thiamin deficiency causes Berberi, a dysfunction of the nervous system. Food sources include whole grain products, pork and pork products, legumes and peas. Thiamin is evenly distributed in foods, however, it is easily destroyed during food processing. Mild thiamin deficiencies are most likely seen in consumers whose diets contain large amounts of food low in nutrients and high in calories, sugar, fat and salt (processed foods).

Niacin

Niacin is necessary for healthy tissues. A deficiency in Niacin will cause Pellagra which was once very common in the United States. The symptoms include rough skin, mouth sores, diarrhea, and mental disorders.

Niacin is very stable and found in foods like liver, lean meat, enriched breads and cereals, whole-grain products, peas and fish.

Vitamin B$_2$ — Riboflavin

Riboflavin helps the body obtain energy from carbohydrates and protein foods. A deficiency of this vitamin causes lip sores and cracks, as well as dimness of vision. Riboflavin is abundant in leafy vegetables, enriched and whole-grains, liver, cheese, lean meats and milk.

Pantothenic Acid

Pantothenic acid is needed to support a variety of body functions including proper growth and maintenance. Symptoms of a deficiency may include headaches, fatigue, poor muscle coordination, nausea, and cramps. Pantothenic acid is found in foods like liver, eggs, white potatoes, sweet potatoes, peas, and whole-grain products.

Folic Acid

Folic acid is essential for the body to manufacture red blood cells and for normal metabolism. A deficiency causes a type of anemia. Folic acid deficiency is the most wide-spread deficiency in the world. Food sources include: dark leafy green vegetables, liver, navy beans, nuts, oranges, and whole-wheat products.

Vitamin B$_6$ — Pyridoxine

This vitamin is part of more than 60 enzyme systems that help regulate nitrogen metabolism. It is also involved with maintaining proper growth and maintenance. Deficiency symptoms include mouth soreness, dizziness, nausea, weight loss, and sometimes severe nervous disturbances.

It has been touted by nutrition quacks for cures of pre-menstrual syndrome (PMS), however, several women who tried megadosing with this vitamin to cure their PMS symptoms came down with severe nervous disorders that have yet to be reversed even though they have been off of the supplements.

Food sources include liver, whole-grain breads and cereal, potatoes, red meats, green vegetables, and yellow corn.

Vitamin B$_{12}$

This vitamin is necessary for the normal development of red blood cells. A deficiency causes pernicious anemia and, if the deficiency is prolonged, a degeneration of the spinal cord occurs.

Abundant sources are organ meats, lean meats, fish, milk, eggs and shellfish. B$_{12}$ is essentially found only in animal food sources and is not present to any measurable degree in plants, which means that strict vegetarians might need to supplement their diets with this vitamin.

Biotin

This vitamin plays an important role in the metabolism of carbohydrates, protein and fats. Some symptoms of deficiency include mild skin disorders, some anemia, depression, sleepiness, and muscle pain. Deficiencies are extremely rare. Food sources include eggs, milk, and meats.

Vitamin C

Most people think of vitamin C's role as only preventing scurvy or helping fight infections, however, vitamin C promotes growth and tissue repair, and aids in tooth and bone formation. The signs and symptoms of vitamin C deficiencies include lassitude, weakness, bleeding, loss of weight, and irritability. Earliest signs of vitamin C deficiencies are bleeding gums and bruising easily. Abundant food sources are turnip greens, green peppers, kale, broccoli, mustard greens, citrus fruits, strawberries, tomatoes, and other vegetables.

Vitamin D

Vitamin D aids in the absorption of calcium and phosphorus for bone formation. Vitamin D is actually not a vitamin in the true sense because it acts like a hormone in the body to help with bone formation. A vitamin D deficiency causes rickets. The obvious signs are skeleton deformations such as bowed legs, deformed spine, and a pot belly appearance.

Vitamin D is the most toxic of all the vitamins. Too much can cause nausea, weight loss, weakness, excessive urination, and a serious problem with calcification of bones. It is ironic that many of the symptoms of toxicity are the same as with a deficiency.

Abundant sources are fish, egg yolks, and fortified milk; however, we get all the vitamin D we need through exposure to ultraviolet sun rays. Athletes who spend part of their training in the sun need no other food source.

Vitamin K

Vitamin K is an essential part of the protein used in the body for blood clotting. Obviously if athletes do not consume enough vitamin K they have problems forming clots. About 50% of the vitamin K you need comes from diet and the other 50% is produced by the bacteria found in your intestines. Vitamin K is found in spinach, lettuce, kale, cabbage, cauliflower, liver, and egg yolks.

Vitamin E

This particular vitamin is receiving a lot of press right now due to its antioxidant role. Vitamin E is a preservative, protecting the activity of other compounds such as vitamin A. No clinical effects have been associated with low levels of vitamin E. A diet high in polyunsaturated fats, including fish oils containing omega 3 fatty acids, may require a small increase in vitamin E due to the fact that free radicals are produced from polyunsaturated fats. Abundant food sources include vegetable oils, beans, eggs, whole grains, liver, some fruits, and vegetables.

While the definitive study has not been done yet to prove that active individuals should be consuming more vitamin E, it would be safe to recommend that you can get all the vitamin E you need by making wise food choices.

Vitamin Cautions

A balanced nutrient supplement providing vitamins in levels at or close to the RDA's has never been shown to be harmful, although nutritionists differ in their opinions as to whether or not these are needed. A caution is clearly in order regarding large intakes of single vitamin supplements, however. High doses of the fat-soluble vitamins A and D can be toxic since the body has no way to effectively excrete them. Table 5.1 lists the vitamins, their functions, what foods they are found in, and potential problems.

PROTECTING THE NUTRIENTS IN YOUR FOOD

Certain vitamins are easily destroyed during food preparation and cooking, so some uncooked servings each day are recommended. A few additional guidelines can assure that you get the most from the foods you buy:

- Store fruits and vegetables in the refrigerator. Warm temperatures speed up natural enzyme processes that break down vitamins once food is harvested.
- Keep fruits and vegetables from being exposed to the air and wrap cut surfaces before storing to preserve vitamin C.
- Slice fruits and vegetables as close to cooking or serving time as possible. Leaving broccoli chopped and sitting on the cutting board for 15 minutes results in large amounts of vitamin C lost.
- Boiling vegetables results in loss of water-soluble nutrients into the water. This cooking water can be refrigerated for later use in soups and sauces, but steaming vegetables avoids much of this loss. If you boil vegetables, cut them in large pieces rather than small pieces. Boil potatoes in their skins.
- Buy fresh and frozen fruits and vegetables rather than canned to obtain the highest amount of nutrients available.
- Vitamin A is destroyed by air and light: riboflavin is destroyed by light. Buy milk in cartons rather than glass bottles if the grocery store dairy case is exposed to light.

MINERALS

Minerals are as basic as chemicals get. They are atoms of inorganic elements. They are not destroyed. They come from the earth's surface, are absorbed by the plant's roots, and incorporated into the structure of the plants. We eventually eat the plants, and they become part of our own body's structure.

Minerals play a specific part of the regulatory mechanism and enzyme system in the body. They also regulate fluid balance, transport substances throughout the body, allow muscles to contract, and nerves to transmit signals as well as perform countless other functions.

Table 5.1. The functions, sources, and potential problems of vitamins.

Vitamin	Function	Best Source	Comments
A	Vision, skin, bone growth, reproduction	Deep yellow and orange fruits and vegetables, dark leafy green vegetables, liver	Retinol is toxic in large amounts; beta carotene has a role in cancer prevention
D	Absorption of calcium, bone growth	Sunlight, fish, fortified milk	Toxic in large amounts
E	Protects cells from oxidative damage	Vegetable oils	Low toxicity
K	Blood clotting	Leafy green vegetables	Synthesized by bacteria in the intestines, deficiencies are rare
C	Connective tissue, wound healing	Citrus fruit, potatoes, leafy veggies, tomatoes	Role in cancer prevention, potential kidney stones from toxic doses
Thiamin (B_1)	Release of energy from carbohydrates	Grains, legumes, pork	
Riboflavin (B_2)	Release of energy from protein, fat and carbohydrate	Dairy products, enriched cereal or whole grains, organ meats, lean meats	Destroyed by exposure to light
Niacin	Release of energy from protein, fat and carbohydrate, synthesis of protein, fat, and DNA	Liver, lean meat, poultry, enriched grains, legumes	Excessive amounts cause liver damage
Pyridoxine (B_6)	Protein synthesis	Whole grains, red meat, eggs, vegetables, liver	Deficiency most common in people whose diets are high in processed food.
Folic Acid	Synthesis of DNA, RNA	Green veggies, liver, legumes, whole grains	Deficiency causes anemia
Vitamin (B_{12})	Aids folacin in DNA	Meat, fish, eggs, cheese, milk, liver	Deficiency anemia synthesis
Pantothenic	Release of energy nutrients	Whole grains, vegetables, fish, poultry, liver	Acid from fuel synthesis of many compounds

Like vitamins, minerals can perform their function repeatedly and at lightening speed. To perform this as well as numerous other tasks, only a few milligrams of minerals are needed in the diet each day; a speck, barely visible to the eye, is hardworking yet essential for life. Table 5.2 lists the major minerals, their food sources, and role in the body.

A couple of minerals seem to be problematic for athletes, especially female athletes.

Table 5.2. Minerals.

Mineral	Function	Best Source	Comments
Calcium	Muscle contractions, blood clotting, bones and teeth	Milk, cheese, leafy greens, fish with bones	Deficiency is Osteoporosis which is common in women
Phosphorus	Bones and teeth, DNA, enzyme reactions	Meat, and other protein foods, soft drinks	Excess contributes to poor bone health
Magnesium	Muscle action, heartbeat, enzyme reaction	Whole grains, molasses	Found in hard water; mild deficiency may be common in diets with alot of processed foods
Sodium	Acid-base balance, fluid balance, muscle action, nerve transmission	Salt, snack foods, cured meats, processed and pickled foods	Excessive intake linked to hypertension
Potassium	Acid-base balance, enzyme reactions	Fruits, especially bananas, molasses	Mild deficiency may contribute to hypertension
Iron	Oxygen transportation in red blood cells	Red meats, grains, liver, prunes, dark leafy greens	Iron deficiency is common among women
Zinc	Role in numerous enzyme reactions	Seafood, meat, whole grains, eggs, nuts	Excessive amounts impair copper, iron, and calcium
Iodine	Component of thyroid	Iodized salt, seafood	
Chromium	Helps aid insulin	Whole grains, molasses, mushrooms, wheat germ	Deficiency may contribute to adult-onset diabetes
Selenium	Component of antioxidant enzymes	Grains, meat, milk, and milk products	Amount depends on soil. Narrow range between safe and toxic amounts

Calcium

The need for calcium is greater during adolescence than during either childhood or adulthood. Approximately 45% of an adult's skeleton mass is formed during the pubescent growth spurt. The RDA of calcium for females aged 11 to 24 years of age is 1,200 milligrams per day. If calcium intake is inadequate during peak bone mass growth, it may predispose the athlete to osteoporosis later in life. Consumption of low-fat dairy products that are rich in calcium should be encouraged. There are many ways to incorporate calcium-rich foods into a diet to meet the daily requirement. For example, two glasses of skim milk and two ounces of low-fat mozzarella cheese contain the recommended dietary allowance for growing adolescent athletes. To incorporate more calcium into your diet, try the tips found in Table 5.3.

Iron

Iron is present in all cells of the body and plays a key role in numerous reactions. It plays a vital role in the transport and activation of oxygen, and is present in several pathways that create energy. Various studies have found the diets of female athletes to be low in iron. One of the problems associated with dieting and limiting calories is that female athletes may not be able to meet their iron requirements. Because females face a greater chance of having low-iron stores, due to the limited calorie intake and increased iron loss through menstruation, it has been suggested that female athletes consider routine use of iron supplements, particularly during periods of heavy training. Iron supplementation, however, in a **non-anemic** female athlete has not been shown to be useful, and may even be harmful. Iron supplementation, taken in excess of the body's need, may lead to increased free radical formation and a condition called hemochromatosis, a disorder where increased iron absorption and deposition in the liver tissue could result in eventually poisoning the liver.

Table 5.3. Increasing calcium in the diet.

- Prepare canned soup with skim milk instead of water
- Add nonfat dry milk to soups, stews, casseroles, and even cookie recipes
- Add grated low-fat mozzarella cheese to salads, tacos, or pasta dishes
- Have yogurt as a snack, or use it to make low-calorie salad dressing and vegetable dip
- Choose calcium-rich desserts such as low-fat cheese, fruit, frozen or low-fat or nonfat yogurt, and puddings made with skim milk
- Drink hot chocolate made with skim milk

Routine screening tests should be performed on prospective female athletes to detect early stages of iron deficiency. Those athletes found to be iron deficient or anemic should receive dietary counseling. Supplemental iron may be indicated in individual cases; however, routine use of iron supplementation by all female athletes is not warranted. To see if you are consuming enough iron, use Table 5.4. Table 5.5 will give you suggestions on how to incorporate more iron into your diet.

Table 5.4. Do you get enough iron?

Food	Serving Size	Iron (mg per serving)
beef liver	3 oz.	4.0
oysters	4	3.6
chicken liver	3 oz.	3.2
pork roast	3 oz.	3.2
roast beef	3 oz.	3.1
leg of lamb	3 oz.	1.9
fillet of sole	3 oz.	1.4
chicken breast	1	1.3
egg	1	1.3
navy beans, cooked	1 cup	5.0
black-eyed peas, cooked	1 cup	4.8
green peas	1 cup	2.9
spinach, cooked	½ cup	2.1
potato, baked	1	1.1
kale, cooked	½ cup	.9
collard greens, cooked	½ cup	.8
broccoli, cooked	½ cup	.6
40% bran flakes	1 cup	12.0
whole wheat bread	1 slice	1.5
rice	½ cup	.5
macaroni, enriched	½ cup	.6
oatmeal	½ cup	.7
prune juice	1 cup	10.5
prunes, cooked	½ cup	2.1
strawberries	1 cup	1.5
molasses	1 tbsp.	3.2

RDA for females age 15-50: 15 mg; females age 51 and older: 10 mg.
RDA for males age 15-18: 12 mg; males age 19 and older: 10 mg.

Meeting a woman's iron need:

4 slices of whole wheat bread	6.0
½ cup beans	2.5
lean beef, 3 ounces	3.1
baked potato	1.1
strawberries, 1 cup	1.5
½ cup of oatmeal	.7
½ cup broccoli	.6
	15.5 mg.

Table 5.5. Increasing iron consumption.

- At each meal, eat foods that are high in Vitamin C to help the body absorb iron. For example, drink orange juice with an iron-fortified cereal, or combine pasta with broccoli and tomatoes.
- Include lean red meats as part of your training diet. These foods provide the body with a form of iron called heme iron. This form is more readily absorbed than the type of iron found in vegetables and grains (non-heme).
- To enhance the absorption of non-heme iron combine vegetable irons with meat. For example, split pea soup with lean ham, tuna-noodle casserole, turkey vegetable soup, or chili beans with ground turkey or lean ground beef.
- To increase iron as well as carbohydrates, eat cereals, breads and pastas that have the words "enriched or fortified" on the labels. Iron is added to these foods during manufacturing.

Mineral Caution

As few as 6 to 12 iron tablets can kill a young child. If you are taking iron supplements and have small children in the house, put them where they can not get to them. Symptoms of intoxication include nausea, vomiting, diarrhea, a rapid heartbeat, a weak pulse, dizziness, shock and confusion. **Among children, iron poisoning deaths are second only to poisonings from aspirin overdose.**

SHOULD ATHLETES TAKE VITAMIN AND MINERAL SUPPLEMENTS?

The greatest interest in vitamin supplementation lies in the perceived potential to supercharge the normal metabolic processes when supplied in amounts greater than those provided in a typical diet. For example, at the International Center for Aquatic Research, elite swimmers were asked in a survey if they felt like they needed to take a supplement. 52% said yes, while 48% said no. When asked in the same survey if they take a supplement, 63% said yes, while 37% said no. While some swimmers felt that they didn't need to take a supplement, some of them were taking a daily vitamin and mineral supplement. Asked why, the response was "just in case" and "the best swimmer on the team is taking it and therefore if I want to be the best I had better take it too." Alot of them were taking vitamin C mainly because they believed that it helped prevent colds. One swimmer who was 14 years of age wrote that he takes 2400 mg of vitamin C every **2 hours** when he feels a cold coming on. He was advised to cut back on the vitamin C if he wanted his kidneys by the time he was 18. Alot of the swimmers were taking individual nutrients like vitamin B_6 without any rationale.

They had just heard that it was suppose to improve their performance. One swimmer was even taking RNA and DNA orally to see if he could change his genetic make-up so that he could swim fast!

There have been years of research undertaken testing the performance effects of acute or chronic intakes of additional vitamins. The results from these numerous studies conclude that supplementation of well-nourished athletes does not appear to improve performance and, therefore, might be considered unnecessary. Athletes who are not eating adequate diets may require specific vitamin and mineral supplements, however, supplements should only be taken under the supervision of a physician or health care professional. Some athletes frequently take iron supplements, believing the extra iron will improve delivery of oxygen to the muscles and, therefore, improve performance. However, if an athlete's diet is supplying adequate amounts of iron, a supplement will not improve performance. Furthermore, taking unnecessary amounts of iron may result in iron overload, which increases the production of free radicals, and large doses of iron can have toxic side effects. Taking excessive amounts of any vitamin or mineral does not improve performance, and there are some vitamins and minerals, which when taken in large doses, can be toxic. If you feel like you need to take a supplement, the recommendation is to take a supplement that has 50-100% of the RDA and perhaps taking it every other day or every 3rd day as opposed to every day. That way you reduce your risk of taking too much of a good thing.

Remember, making half-way decent food choices will provide you with all the vitamins and minerals your body needs even when you are training hard.

6 Nutritional Ergogenic Aids

> "Quackery has no such friend as credulity."
> —C. Simmons

INTRODUCTION

As long as competitive sports have existed, athletes have attempted to improve their performance by ingesting a variety of nutritional supplements. At one time it was believed that eating certain foods would impart desirable characteristics on the person who ate them. Consequently, some athletes would eat the meat of a bull before competition in an effort to increase strength and courage. From drinking elexirs in ancient Greece to modern-day carbohydrate beverages, athletes have used different substances to improve performance or reverse their body's fatigue.

The term, ergogenic aid, is defined as a work-enhancing aid. Any substance, technique or piece of equipment used in an effort to improve performance may be considered an ergogenic aid. The most often used and abused ergogenic aids, however, are nutritional ergogenic aids. Pick up any health and fitness magazine, and you can hardly turn a page without seeing an advertisement for a new product or compound "hyped" to improve performance.

Athletes have a burning desire for the answers to questions like these:

- Do substances such as supplements derived from plant sterols (cholesterol and its derivatives, including steroid hormones and various vitamins) provide as much as 50 percent of the biological activity of anabolic steroids?
- Will the mineral boron promote testosterone synthesis in the body?
- Will royal jelly (produced by worker bees and fed to the queen bee) benefit endurance performance?
- Will carnitine increase my weight loss?

In each case there is virtually no scientific research to support the claims of these products.

In 1992, the National Council Against Health Fraud's Task Force on Ergogenic Aids published an article called "Deceptive Tactics Used in Marketing Purported Ergogenic Aids" in the *National Strength and Conditioning Association Journal*. They reviewed claims made by 45 companies that sell ergogenic aids and outlined practices they believe to be unacceptable. Here are the nine points that were highlighted in that article:

1) Misrepresentation of research. Research is taken out of context, or unmerited conclusions are referred to it. "University tested" may imply only that someone inside a university was involved, with no evidence of whether the study had merit. Implied endorsement by teams may mean that the company sent the team samples, and they were not sent back.
2) "We are currently doing double blind research" is common statement, but rarely true.
3) "Research not for public review" thwarts the consumer's right to documentation of performance claims.
4) Testimonials. Even a placebo will produce results in some people that will make them believe its effectiveness.
5) Patents. A patent says nothing about the effectiveness of a product.
6) Inappropriately used research. Research that is poorly controlled, outdated, taken out of context, not peer reviewed, or from Eastern European sources cannot be relied upon.
7) Publicity and articles planted in publications to avoid possible prosecution for the same false and misleading claims if made in an ad.
8) Mail-order evaluations. Computerized evaluations conveniently find that the consumer needs the products the company wants to sell.
9) Anabolic measurements based on nitrogen balance. These don't correlate to increased lean body mass, so do not prove the worth of very high protein supplements.

It's okay to be a skeptic. In fact, it's your responsibility. Question claims, especially ones that seem too good to be true. Remember, just because something appears in print, does not mean that it's true.

Ten Questions That Put Supplements to the Test

Below are 10 questions to ask when purchasing a nutritional supplement, evaluating their advertising or literature.

1) What scientific evidence is available to support the claim?
2) Where were the scientific studies conducted?
3) By whom? What were the researchers' and laboratories' qualifications?

4) Do the researchers have commercial or financial interest in the company?
5) Where was the study published? Was it a reputable scientific journal or a magazine?
6) Was the study peer reviewed?
7) Are there any other studies to support or deny the claims?
8) What do recognized experts in the field say about the research?
9) Who are the experts? What are their credentials?
10) Do the experts have financial interest in the product?

Table 6.1. Some of the more popular nutritional ergogenic aids used by athletes.

Ergogenic Aid	Description	Claim
Ginseng	Extract of ginseng root	Adaptogen —protection against tissue
Inosine	Enhances physical strength	
Carnitine	A compound synthesized in the body from amino acids	Helps transport fats into muscle cells
Bee pollen	Mixture of bee pollen	Increased energy levels
Lecithin	Prevents fat gain	
Kelp	Seaweed	Source of vitamins and minerals
Royal jelly	Produced by worker bee and fed to Queen bee	Increased strength
Spirulina	Blue-green algae	Source of protein
Smilax	Increase blood testosterone levels	
Brewer's Yeast	By-product of beer brewing	Increased energy levels
Octacosanol	Extracted from wheat germ	Increased endurance

LEGAL PERFORMANCE ENHANCERS

Are there any nutritional supplements that are potentially promising? Recent research studies have suggested that ingesting creatine and bicarbonate may enhance high-intensity performance. Other studies have shown that large doses of caffeine may increase endurance. These and other nutritional supplements that have been put through scientific testing to substantiate their benefits in athletic performance will now be discussed in further detail.

Creatine Loading: A Safe and Legal Way to Faster Times?

Scientists are claiming a major breakthrough with a new food compound which could eradicate drugs from sport and herald a crop of world records. The substance, creatine, is a muscle fuel occurring naturally in meat and fish which has been developed in tablet and capsule forms by several supplement companies. Creatine will allow you to train harder, longer, and raises energy levels for explosive events such as sprints in running or bicycling. The good news for endurance athletes is that its benefits may not be limited to sprinters.

Your liver produces creatine naturally — about two grams every day — from glycine and arginine, two nonessential amino acids. The creatine is then transported in your blood to your heart, skeletal muscles, and other body cells. In the muscles, creatine is used to form creatine phosphate (CP), a high-powered chemical, which supplies the energy needed for muscles to keep contracting in sprints lasting approximately 10 to 15 seconds. CP is used to rebuild the ultimate energy source of your muscles' adenosine triphosphate (ATP). This is an extremely rapid reaction, and since the CP concentration can fall to almost zero, it allows your muscles to perform high-intensity exercise for only short periods. As a result, for maximum performance in power and sprint events an athlete who can supplement their muscles with CP will be at an advantage.

CP is also used during intermediate anaerobic (15 seconds to several minutes) work where the break down of CP will help buffer the increased intracellular acidity caused by lactic acid buildup. More CP in the muscle cell means greater buffering capacity within the cell and, therefore, a greater resistance to fatigue. Increased levels of CP could help in events requiring intermittent bursts of speed or sustained anaerobic work, such as 5 kilometer runs, soccer or basketball.

Lastly, CP is used to help with the transfer of energy within the muscle cell. During aerobic work ATP is produced in large quantities within the mitochondria where fats, protein and carbohydrates are broken down to produce ATP, but it must be transferred to the contractile proteins. This transfer process requires an adequate supply of CP, and an increased CP content within the cell may make the action more rapid. In events such as marathons or triathlons, if creatine is increased in the muscle cell it may help make the process more rapid.

Among those to already use creatine and having made public statements in the *London Times* are British athletes, Linford Christie and Sally Gunnell, who won gold medals in the 1992 Olympic Games. It was also reported in several newspapers from informed sources that during the games Bulgarian weight lifters and Russian soccer players may have been supplementing their diet with creatine. But it is not just athlete testimonials that are showing coaches, athletes and scientists that creatine is a powerful ergogenic aid. Several studies in humans and horses (thoroughbred racers and harness racers) showed that creatine supplements increased performance and recovery time.

Recent studies in human sports science have shown that supplementation of the normal diet with creatine will increase its content in the muscles. A study published in a 1992 issue of *Clinical Science* showed when the diets of individuals were supplemented several times per day that muscle creatine concentrations were increased by over 35 percent in exercising muscles. This work was completed by Dr. Eric Hultman, who in the early 1960's produced the original research on the importance of carbohydrate loading in increasing time to fatigue during endurance exercise. Today, he is showing that creatine supplementation can help increase an athlete's performance times in sprint events.

In a similar study recently reported at a scientific conference, Dr. Hultman and other researchers supplemented five middle distance runners with creatine over a 6-day period while another group received a placebo supplementation for the same time period. Prior to and following the 6-days of supplementation, the runners ran four 1,000-meter intervals on one day and four 300-meter sprints on another day. Compared to the placebo group, after supplementation the creatine group times to run four 1,000-meter intervals decreased from 769.8 seconds to 757 seconds, while the placebo group's time was actually slowed from 774.1 seconds to 775. 3 seconds. For the 300-meter sprints the times for the placebo groups decreased from 41.7 to 41.4 seconds, and the creatine supplemented group dropped from 38.4 to 37.7 seconds. The creatine group had statistically significant decreases in times at both distances.

A 1994 issue of the *Penn State Sports Medicine Newsletter* reported on a study in which eight Swedish physical education students were given creatine supplements for five days, while another group of eight subjects was given a placebo substance. After five days, the subjects performed sprints on a stationary bicycle at 130-pedal revolutions per minute for 10 seconds with 30 seconds rest between sprints. The next day the test was repeated, this time with the pedal revolutions raised to 140 trying to induce fatigue more quickly.

The creatine group was able to maintain a higher pedaling rate over the final few seconds of each sprint bout, while the placebo group decreased their power output in the final moments of each sprint. In addition to increased power output in the creatine group, these subjects also had lower blood lactic acid accumulations even though they were doing more work.

In addition subjective, but scientifically unsubstantiated reports indicate that recovery from intense activity may be faster following supplementation, and that in trained subjects the incidence of post-exercise muscle stiffness is reduced.

Vegetarians also have much to gain from creatine supplementation. Their diets are void of creatine, and they tend to have lower levels of blood and urine creatine. In fact, in Hultman's first study, one of the runners who was a vegetarian increased creatine muscle content by approximately 60 percent, compared to the group mean of 35 percent.

Now you are probably asking how much food would I need to consume to increase my muscle creatine levels enough to have an ergogenic affect? You would probably have to eat between 5 and 6 pounds of beef per day. Since this is highly unlikely, creatine supplementation by tablet form is the only reasonable way to accomplish the levels needed for improved performance.

Currently, there are several commercial sources of creatine supplements since it has been permitted to be sold by the U. S. Food and Drug Administration. Most suppliers suggest a maintenance dose of creatine of about 2 grams per day, and a loading regimen of 9 to 10 grams per day for the last week before a major competition. Just as with carbohydrate loading, you would only follow the loading regimen 3 to 4 times per year. In theory, with your muscles now supersaturated with creatine, there would be more creatine phosphate for explosive exercise.

There have been no significant side effects reported in the few studies that have been in the literature. And because excess creatine is excreted in your urine, the use of creatine in supplement form of about 2 grams, at this time, does not appear to pose a medical risk. However, anyone taking over 30 grams or more per day, as used in some of the research studies for extended periods of time, should be monitored by their physician for possible liver or kidney damage.

Creatine supplementation is a new concept in sports nutrition. The aim of creatine supplements is to meet the specific nutritional needs of muscles in the quest to raise performance potential of the athlete. Since creatine is a legitimate food supplement which supplies large amounts of fuel to your muscles, it's not banned by any sport's national governing body or the International Olympic Committee. From the scientific research and anecdotal evidence of athletes, it appears that creatine is a legal ergogenic aid that works. And like carbohydrate loading, creatine may be routine for anyone training hard and competing.

Caffeine: A Stimulating Topic For Sports Performance

In his popular book *Eat To Win*, Robert Hass states that "caffeine provides endurance athletes with an unquestionable, scientifically demonstrable advantage over opponents of roughly equal athletic ability." This and other statements in the popular press have convinced multi-sport athletes that ingesting caffeine will improve performance. But what dose of caffeine is necessary to gain an ergogenic effect? And, when is its use justified in sports?

Caffeine is one of a group of compounds called methylxanthines that occur naturally in over 60 species of plants, including coffee beans, cocoa beans, cola nuts and tea leaves. It is, thus, naturally present in coffee, tea, cola soft drinks, cocoa and chocolate. The amount of caffeine per serving varies with the type of product. The caffeine content per five-ounce cup is about 60-150 mg for drip or percolated coffee, 40-110 mg for instant coffee, 2-5 mg for decaffeinated coffee, 10-50 mg for brewed tea and 10-30 mg for instant tea. Soft drinks range from 0-60 mg of caffeine per 12-ounce serving.

Caffeine also serves a variety of pharmacological functions and is found in combination with drugs used as stimulants, cold remedies, pain remedies, diuretics and weight-control products.

Caffeine stimulates the central nervous system and can reduce a variety of effects elsewhere in the body. Depending on the dose, caffeine can increase metabolic rate, heart rate and step up the production of urine. Caffeine also affects the central nervous system by enhancing perception, alertness and possibly reducing fatigue during muscular work.

Caffeine has received mixed reviews in research studies looking at increased performance. In athletes, the primary findings have focused on the ability of caffeine to increase endurance. It increases fat metabolism by raising the levels of free fatty acids in the blood, which means that your stores of fat are used for energy production, rather than limited stores of carbohydrates (glycogen). Caffeine prolongs endurance by enhancing fat use and sparing glycogen depletion. When released into the blood from body stores, fat — of which there is almost always an ample supply (even in highly-trained athletes) — can power your body's muscles during prolonged running, cycling or swimming.

While many scientists question the ability of caffeine to improve performance outside of laboratory research, a recent "field" research study has shown that caffeine can help in actual race conditions. The study was conducted at Christ Church College in England, and asked 18 runners of various levels of ability to run a 1500-meter time trial on two separate occasions. In one trial they ran after drinking two cups of strong coffee containing 150 to 200 mg of caffeine each, and the other run was completed following two cups of decaffeinated coffee. Of the 18 runners, 14 of them ran on the average of 4 seconds faster after drinking the caffeinated coffee — which was also found to be statistically significant.

In a second test of caffeine's effect upon performance, 10 runners were asked to "sprint" the final 400 meters of a 1500-meter time trial. In this trial the runners were asked to cover the first 1100 meters at a fixed pace, and then sprint the final 400 meters. All 10 runners ran the final 400 meters faster after consuming caffeine and also had lower blood lactic acid levels. The researchers concluded that the caffeine improved muscular power and reduced the mental sense of exercise fatigue.

While the majority of research extols the use of caffeine, several studies have found caffeine to have no effect. This probably means that everyone is different, and the dosage of caffeine needed to improve performance is unknown.

Caffeine has some detrimental effects. Caffeine is a powerful diuretic (as is apparent from the inevitable need to visit the bathroom after a coffee break). This can be a serious problem in hot weather, where hydration is imperative. Some athletes also complain of nausea when caffeine is used in hot weather.

There are mixed opinions among endurance athletes and researchers over the timing and amount of caffeine to ingest to improve performance. For long distance events, drinking about one to two cups of coffee 45-60 minutes before the race, and ingesting some caffeine periodically during the race, seems to be the recommended practice to increase performance. The amount of caffeine you ingest is crucial. If you ingest too much, you will experience gastric upset and expresso nerves, and you will begin to dehydrate yourself because of excessive urine production. It seems that the dosage of about 5 mg of caffeine per kilogram of body weight (2.2 pounds equals one kilogram) is the appropriate dosage. When people begin to take over 7 mg per kilogram of body weight, they start to get headaches and do not feel well. One should bear in mind, though, that caffeine affects everyone differently.

Some scientists have stated that the difference between taking caffeine (coffee, cola, Vivarin, No-Doz) and amphetamines in competition is a matter of ethics. A similar matter of ethics could be questioned in the use of carbohydrate loading or excessive vitamin supplements. These also can be considered forms of doping. To make matters worse, the International Olympic Committee has been changing its mind on the matter of caffeine for years. At one time it was illegal, then for a period of time it was legal, and then levels of over 15 micrograms (mcg) of caffeine per milliliter (ml) of urine became grounds for disqualification. Now the level has been changed again, and an amount greater than 12 mcg/ml is considered doping. As an example, to reach this limit one would have to consume approximately six to eight cups of coffee in one sitting and be tested within two to three hours. However, there are other sources of caffeine, such as colas, aspirin, and Vivarin that may cause excessive levels in the urine. During the course of a day's competition, an athlete may inadvertently take in too much caffeine and show up positive on testing.

Caffeine is a legal nutritional supplement, and athletes are free to experiment with it. But caution must be exercised. While it most likely will increase endurance performance, its improper use could have detrimental side effects. Lastly, caffeine's improper use could lead to disqualification in competition.

Chromium

If you have been following the nutritional scene, you know that the use of chromium supplements has increased in the past few years. Many magazines are promoting chromium as a safe alternative to anabolic steroids. They promote the idea that chromium will increase muscle mass without the adverse effects of steroids.

There are two possible ways that the mineral chromium could increase muscle mass. Chromium links together chains of amino acids to form proteins, so it's possible that extra chromium may help increase muscle growth by stimulating protein production. By increasing the influx of amino acids into muscle cells and directing the synthesis of new protein from these amino acids can increase muscle mass.

While most athletes may not be interested in increasing muscle mass, protein synthesis may be important in the amount of time needed to recover from a tough workout. For instance, it may take several days to recover after a hard race; if you can recover quicker, your training could be re-initiated earlier. Protein is important for the repair of microtrauma to muscles, ligaments and tendons.

The mineral also serves to facilitate the activity of insulin. Insulin promotes the uptake of glucose by the muscles and promotes glycogen storage, and without chromium, insulin itself cannot work. Although the exact mechanism in which the mineral interacts with insulin is not known, based upon the work of its co-discoverer, Dr. Walter Mertz, it appears that chromium improves the attachment of insulin to the receptors on the surface of the insulin cells. The net result is that chromium makes insulin much more efficient. In other words, it could aid in carbohydrate loading.

The recommended daily amount of chromium is small, 50 to 200 mcg. That's about 1/28 millionth of an ounce of chromium daily. However, there is no test available to you that will show if you are chromium deficient.

Even so, the average male takes in about 33 mcg of chromium a day and the average female takes in about 25 mcg. Habits or dietary deficiencies that may make you chromium deficient include:

- Eating lots of sugar, which tends to increase urinary chromium excretion.
- Stress and heavy exercise increase your need for chromium.
- Eating lots of refined foods and white flour, for these foods are low in chromium content.

If you practice two or more of the above, you may want to consider changing your diet or taking chromium supplements. Foods which are good sources of chromium are: Brewer's yeast, mushrooms, whole grains, apples and shellfish. Before you consider taking a supplement, be aware that there are several types of chromium on the market. Chromium picolinate, polynicotinate, and other trivalent forms of chromium are the common forms found in supplements and are absorbed much better than inorganic forms of chromium supplements.

The scientific literature suggests that large doses of chromium could lead to malabsorption of zinc and iron, leading to possible deficiencies in those minerals. Several medical authorities also point to possible pancreatic damage, which will affect insulin production.

While there is some scientific and dietary evidence that chromium deficiencies exist in some of our diets and that it may improve performance, there is still lots to learn about this mineral. Taking chromium supplements at the estimated and safe levels appears to have no adverse effects.

Soda Loading

Soda loading — the ingestion of sodium bicarbonate, plain old baking soda, to neutralize the buildup of lactic acid in muscles and reduce fatigue — has never been banned as an ergogenic aid. During strenuous activity, your body produces an excess of lactic acid which builds up in the blood and muscle cells. This increased acidity ultimately contributes to muscle fatigue. Increasing the sodium bicarbonate concentration in the blood can help buffer or neutralize lactic acid by causing it to leave muscle cells and enter the blood more rapidly than normal. Less lactic acid in your muscles equals less fatigue.

The usual dosage of sodium bicarbonate administrated is about 0.30 grams/kg of body weight taken about 1 to 2 hours prior to the exercise. It is usually taken over a 30-minute period and is consumed in gelatin capsules or dissolved in fluid. If capsules are used, it is important to drink approximately one liter of water to minimize gastrointestinal distress.

Unfortunately, the research investigating the effects of bicarbonate loading have produced conflicting results. Several studies show that performance in short-term exercise (30 to 100 seconds) is not improved by the ingestion of sodium bicarbonate. Lactic acid, however, is probably not the factor causing fatigue in events lasting less than two minutes. On the other hand, several studies have reported performance improvements in events lasting from 2 to 10 minutes and during repeated bouts of interval training.

Much of the controversy brought about by the conflicting results of these studies is based on the following:

1) Bicarbonate loading will have very little affect on sprint or short power events.
2) Bicarbonate ingestion may improve performance in intermediate distance anaerobic events such as cycling, running and swimming.
3) The doses of sodium bicarbonate required to obtain any benefit are so large that severe physical discomfort usually occurs.
4) The timing of bicarbonate doses is nearly impossible to regulate for any specific individual, and several reports show that inappropriate use of sodium bicarbonate can actually be responsible for negative results in competition.

Bicarbonate loading has produced negative results in some athletes. Negative effects that have been reported include: intestinal discomfort and stomach distress, nausea, cramping and diarrhea, and water retention. Anyone who has high blood pressure should not use bicarbonate. In the most severe cases, because of the large shift in blood alkalinity, death could also occur.

Sodium bicarbonate is not currently on the International Olympic Committee (IOC) list of banned substances, although some consider its use a violation of the IOC doping rule that bans the use of any substance taken in an attempt to artificially enhance performance. Although there is no test to detect the use of sodium bicarbonate, an excessively alkaline urine may provide some indication of potential abuses.

Choline

Another trace mineral commanding a lot of attention recently in the layman's press, choline is involved in the neurological processes responsible for muscular contraction. Researchers hypothesize that low levels of this chemical may contribute to the onset of muscular fatigue.

James Wurtman, Ph.D. of the Massachusetts Institute of Technology, studied a group of runners who had just completed the Boston Marathon and found a 40 percent drop in their choline levels. Subsequently, he gave the runners supplements of choline an hour before and then again halfway through a 20-mile run. Sure enough, several of the runners ran an average five minutes faster for the run, having taken the choline supplement.

Wurtman believes that fatigue may be due in large part to low levels of choline, causing less than optimal efficient muscle contraction. As with chromium, more research is needed to confirm the usefulness of choline supplementation.

MCTs: A Fat That Metabolizes Like a Carbohydrate

A fat that is metabolized like a carbohydrate could be a boon to all athletes desiring a high energy food during racing or training. The fat — medium chain triglyceride (MCT) oil — is now sold in health food stores for about $10 a pint and quickly becoming the "energy food" of the 90's.

MCTs are saturated fats that are composed of 6 to 12 carbons, while long chain triglycerides (LCT) are saturated and unsaturated fats with 14 to 24 carbons. Palm oil, cocoa butter, corn oil, dairy fats and tallow are examples of LCTs. Kernel oils and coconut oil contain MCT, with coconut oil containing about 15 percent 8-10 carbon chain fatty acids. MCT oil is essentially 100 percent 8-10 carbon fatty acid triglycerides. MCTs don't naturally occur in nature; they are processed from oils.

MCTs are absorbed differently by the body than regular fats. They are rapidly absorbed and can become a more immediate source of energy (like carbohydrates), but they are not as readily stored as body fat because they burn rapidly. They can be used directly by your liver where they are readily burned as energy. It has also been speculated that MCTs can improve endurance performance because they can enter your mitochondria (the aerobic powerhouse of your muscle cells) easier than LCTs. Your muscles produce most of their energy during exercise by breaking down fat and carbohydrate inside the mitochondria. Since MCTs are able to enter the mitochondria rapidly, they should increase energy production and help to conserve the muscles' stores of carbohydrate.

In addition, unlike carbohydrates, which supply 4 calories per gram, MCTs supply 8.3 calories per gram (slightly less than some other forms of fat). Athletes seeking a ready source can take advantage of MCTs ability to deliver more calories per gram than carbohydrates.

Until recently, scientists have only speculated on how MCTs may have improved your performance. That all changed when a group of researchers led by Tim Noakes in South Africa showed improved performance during a 40-kilometer time trial. Six trained cyclists completed three endurance rides on separate days that began with a two-hour ride at about 70 percent of their maximum heart rate. Each ride was then followed by a 40-kilometer time trial during which they were instructed to complete as quickly as possible. During the three rides, the cyclists consumed either a 4.3 percent MCT beverage, a 10 percent carbohydrate beverage or a beverage containing both 4.3 percent MCTs and 10 percent carbohydrate. In all three rides, the cyclists consumed 14 ounces of the drink at the beginning of the ride and then about 3.5 ounces every ten minutes of the ride.

After all the tests were completed the MCT-carbohydrate drink produced the best performance in the 40-kilometer time trial — just 65 minutes, versus 66:45 minutes with carbohydrates, and a slow 72 minutes with just the MCTs.

The researchers suggest that MCTs added to the carbohydrate drink improved performance by decreasing carbohydrate depletion in their legs during the first two hours of the ride, by replacing the carbohydrate as the primary fuel source during the two hours of riding. As a result, when the subjects increased their intensity during the time trial, the combined beverage spared more carbohydrate for the high-intensity effort.

Owen Anderson, in a 1994 issue of *Running Research News*, suggests that a MCT drink alone may conserve glycogen (stored carbohydrate), but it cannot replace carbohydrate that has already been used by the muscles — only a carbohydrate beverage can do that. But a beverage with MCTs and carbohydrates can have a double effect. They can decrease the use of glycogen by the muscles and substitute for the used glycogen. Drinks with only MCTs can only slow glycogen depletion.

Before you run out and start adding MCTs to your sports drink, Owen Anderson points out that MCT-carbohydrate drinks may only be of benefit to road races or training rides lasting more than two or three hours. In shorter events, during which intensities are usually higher, your muscles prefer to only use carbohydrates. It is only during long endurance events that MCTs can be of benefit to performance.

MCT's can be purchased at your local health food store under such labels as ThinOil® (Sound Nutrition) and MCT Fuel® (TwinLab). On your next long ride try mixing your own MCT-carbohydrate drink (a good mix would be 4 to 5 percent MCT and 8 to 10 percent carbohydrate). This would be 4-5 grams of MCTs and 8-10 grams of carbohydrate power in every 100 milliliters (3.4 ounces) of water. If entering an event lasting more than two hours, give this MCT-carbohydrate cocktail a try; you may see dramatic improvement in your performances.

BUYER BEWARE

The bottom line regarding nutritional supplements is caveat emptor — let the buyer beware! Most of us like to believe that we're too well informed to fall for the latest miracle supplement. But when you're training hard and the performance gains are not coming as quickly as you'd like, the temptation to try something in a bottle or capsule is great.

"It's the new steroid substitute." In times of hard training you may look favorably upon such a product claim if a well-placed advertisement suggested that taking such a product may produce gains in muscle mass. But, until proven otherwise, remember that eating a diet high in carbohydrate and training hard are still the best ergogenic aids available. Most supplements should only be used as insurance policies against inadequate diets.

7 Weight Control

"He who does not mind his belly will hardly mind anything else."
—*Samuel Johnson*

INTRODUCTION

Each athlete has a specific requirement for calories. Age, sex, weight and training mileage or yardage determine their caloric needs. The caloric cost of the sport depends on the frequency, intensity, and duration of the activity. The more intense the exercise and the longer it's carried out, the greater the caloric cost. Sedentary individuals require about 30 kcal/kg daily (14 kcal/lb), whereas athletes who train daily require 50 kcal/kg daily (23 kcal/lb) or more.

Maintaining weight, gaining weight, or losing weight is a matter of energy balance. An athlete's body weight will stay the same when caloric intake equals caloric output. It will change when there is an imbalance between caloric intake and caloric expenditure. To gain weight, energy intake must be greater than energy output. To lose weight, energy output must be greater than energy intake. In short, if you need to lose fat weight, you must eat less and exercise more, or both.

BODY COMPOSITION

Many athletes and coaches decide to lose weight based solely on a number they read from a bathroom scales. However, the scale does not differentiate between fat weight and muscle weight. Athletes automatically assume that a gain in scale weight represents a gain of fat weight or that a loss of scale weight is fat loss. There are many situations in which this is not true. For example, an athlete on a training program will probably gain weight; however, the weight gain is due to the addition of muscle mass, not fat.

A scale cannot determine how fat a person is, because both fat and muscle, as well as the skeletal structure and body fluids contribute to total weight. A more accurate indicator of fitness is body composition, which divides weight into two categories. One is lean body mass, which

105

muscle is a major component. The other category is fat mass. What is important, though, is how much of an athlete's weight is fat. This is expressed as percent body fat. It is the percentage of body fat, in conjunction with total body weight, that should determine whether an athlete needs to lose weight.

The athlete who suffers the most, when evaluated by a scale alone, is the stocky muscular type. This type of athlete has very little fat, however, they weigh more than their teammates because of their higher content of lean body mass. Lean body mass weighs more than fat mass, so as a result these athletes have a low percent of body fat and yet weigh more because they have a large component of lean body mass. If they are told to lose weight just because they are stocky (and people perceive that as being overweight), they will have to lose muscle and probably experience a deterioration in their athletic performance. This is just one example of why body composition assessment is so important before initiating a weight-loss program, especially in athletes.

Assessing Body Composition

Underwater Weighing

Hydrostatic weighing at residual volume has become the gold standard or criterion method by which all other indirect, noninvasive methods have been developed and validated. Hydrostatic weighing is based on Archimedes' principle for assessing body volume. Archimedes discovered that the volume of an object can be determined by its loss of weight in water, that is its actual weight minus its weight under water. Knowing the volume of a body and its mass or weight makes it possible to calculate density. The density of the body is then determined through the simple relationship of weight to volume. Once the body density has been assessed from hydrostatic weighing, percentage of body fat can be estimated.

Anthropometric Measurements

Circumferences

Circumference measurements are affected by skin, muscle, fat and bone. Circumferential dimensions of the body, alone or in combination with skinfold measurements, have been used for such indices as fat patterning, muscular development, nutrition assessment, and frame size. Measurements appear to be easy to make, but obtaining accurate and reliable readings can be somewhat difficult. A tape measure should be selected that is flexible but non-elastic and about 0.7 cm wide. The tape should be held firmly but not so tight that the skin is compressed. Except for the neck and head, measurements are taken so that the plane of the tape around the body is perpendicular to the long axis of that body part. Using Table 7.1 you can determine your own percent

Table 7.1. How to measure circumferences. (Courtesy of National Dairy Council®)

One way to find out how much body fat an athlete has is by measuring girths with a tape measure. The circumference method of calculating body fat is relatively accurate, although not as accurate as skinfolds or underwater weighing. Depending on your age and sex, measure athletes at the following places.*

MALES 15 TO 26 YEARS OF AGE
- right upper arm (halfway between the shoulder and the elbow, with the arm straight)
- abdomen (½ inch above the navel)
- right forearm (the widest part between the elbow and wrist)

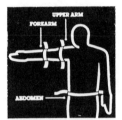

MALES 27 TO 50 YEARS OF AGE
- buttocks (maximum protrusion with heels together)
- abdomen (½ inch above the navel)
- right forearm (the widest part between the elbow and wrist)

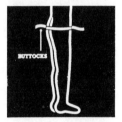

FEMALES 15 TO 26 YEARS OF AGE
- abdomen (½ inch above the navel)
- right thigh (just below the buttocks)
- right forearm (the widest part between the elbow and wrist)

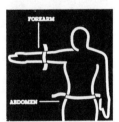

FEMALES 27 TO 50 YEARS OF AGE
- abdomen (½ inch above the navel)
- right thigh (just below the buttocks)
- right calf (the widest part halfway between the ankle and knee)

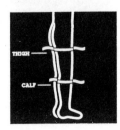

*After measuring an athlete and recording the measurements, change the measurements to constants and calculate the percent body fat using the formulas in the next table.

Adapted from McArdle, Katch and Katch. *Exercise Physiology*. Philadelphia, Pa: Lea and Febiger, 1991.

Table 7.1. (*Continued*)

Calculating constants for body fat using the circumference method for MALES 15 TO 26 YEARS OF AGE.

UPPER ARM		ABDOMEN		RIGHT FOREARM	
Measurement	Constant	Measurement	Constant	Measurement	Constant
7″	26	21″	28	7″	38
8″	30	22″	29	8″	43
9″	33	23″	30	9″	49
10″	37	24″	31	10″	54
11″	41	25″	33	11″	60
12″	44	26″	34	12″	65
13″	48	27″	35	13″	71
14″	52	28″	37	14″	76
15″	56	29″	38	15″	81
16″	59	30″	39	16″	87
17″	63	31″	41	17″	92
18″	67	32″	42	18″	98
19″	70	33″	43	19″	103
20″	74	34″	45	20″	109
21″	78	35″	46	21″	114
22″	81	36″	47	22″	119
		37″	49		
		38″	50		
		39″	51		
		40″	52		
		41″	54		
		42″	55		

Write the **constants** for the measurements in the formula. DO NOT USE THE ACTUAL MEASURE-MENTS IN THIS FORMULA. Then do the necessary addition and subtraction.

Upper arm constant   _____
Abdomen constant   + _____

Subtotal   _____
Forearm constant   = _____

Subtotal   _____
          −10* _____

Approximate body fat   _____ %

*For athletes use 14 instead

Table 7.1. (*Continued*)

Calculating constants for body fat using the circumference method for MALES 27 TO 50 YEARS OF AGE.

BUTTOCKS		ABDOMEN		RIGHT FOREARM	
Measurement	Constant	Measurement	Constant	Measurement	Constant
28″	29	26″	23	7″	21
29″	30	27″	24	8″	24
30″	31	28″	25	9″	27
31″	32	29″	26	10″	30
32″	34	30″	27	11″	33
33″	35	31″	28	12″	36
34″	36	32″	29	13″	39
35″	37	33″	30	14″	42
36″	38	34″	30	15″	45
37″	39	35″	31	16″	48
38″	40	36″	32	17″	51
39″	41	37″	33	18″	54
40″	42	38″	34		
41″	43	39″	35		
42″	44	40″	36		
43″	45	41″	37		
44″	46	42″	38		
45″	47	43″	39		
46″	48	44″	40		
47″	49	45″	40		
48″	50				
49″	51				

Write the ***constants*** for the measurements in the formula. DO NOT USE THE ACTUAL MEASUREMENTS IN THIS FORMULA. Then do the necessary addition and subtraction.

Buttocks
Abdomen constant   + _____

Subtotal
Forearm constant   = _____

Subtotal
    −15* _____

Approximate body fat   _____ %

*For athletes use 19 instead

Table 7.1. (*Continued*)

Calculating constants for body fat using the circumference method for FEMALES 15 TO 26 YEARS OF AGE.

ABDOMEN		RIGHT THIGH		RIGHT FOREARM	
Measurement	Constant	Measurement	Constant	Measurement	Constant
20″	27	14″	29	6″	26
21″	28	15″	31	7″	30
22″	29	16″	33	8″	34
23″	31	17″	35	9″	39
24″	32	18″	37	10″	43
25″	33	19″	40	11″	47
26″	35	20″	42	12″	52
27″	36	21″	44	13″	56
28″	37	22″	46	14″	60
29″	39	23″	48	15″	65
30″	40	24″	50	16″	69
31″	41	25″	52	17″	73
32″	43	26″	54	18″	78
33″	44	27″	56	19″	82
34″	45	28″	58	20″	86
35″	47	29″	60		
36″	48	30″	62		
37″	49	31″	65		
38″	51	32″	67		
39″	52	33″	69		
40″	53	34″	71		

Write the *constants* for the measurements in the formula. DO NOT USE THE ACTUAL MEASUREMENTS IN THIS FORMULA. Then do the necessary addition and subtraction.

Abdomen constant
Thigh constant   +_____

Subtotal   _____
Forearm constant   =_____

Subtotal   _____
                                  –20*_____

Approximate body fat   _____ %

*For athletes use 23 instead

Table 7.1. (*Continued*)

Calculating constants for body fat using the circumference method for FEMALES 27 TO 50 YEARS OF AGE.

ABDOMEN		RIGHT THIGH		RIGHT CALF	
Measurement	Constant	Measurement	Constant	Measurement	Constant
25″	30	14″	17	10″	14
26″	31	16″	19	11″	16
27″	32	17″	20	12″	17
28″	33	18″	21	13″	19
29″	34	19″	22	14″	20
30″	36	20″	23	15″	22
31″	37	21″	24	16″	23
32″	38	22″	26	17″	25
33″	39	23″	27	18″	26
34″	40	24″	28	19″	27
35″	42	25″	29	20″	29
36″	43	26″	31	21″	30
37″	44	27″	32	22″	32
38″	45	28″	33	23″	33
39″	46	29″	35	24″	35
40″	48	30″	36	25″	36
41″	49	31″	37		
42″	50	32″	38		
43″	51	33″	40		
44″	52	34″	41		
45″	53	35″	42		

Write the *constants* for the measurements in the formula. DO NOT USE THE ACTUAL MEASUREMENTS IN THIS FORMULA. Then do the necessary addition and subtraction.

Abdomen constant	_____
Thigh constant	+ _____
Subtotal	_____
Calf constant	= _____
Subtotal	_____
	−18* _____
Approximate body fat	_____ %

*For athletes use 21 instead

body fat by taking your measurements with a tape measure. These measurements are **NOT** 100 percent accurate. But they will give you a good idea of your present level of body fat. The measurements and formulas are based on your age and sex. Use the correct formula to find out your estimated percent body fat.

Skinfolds

Skinfold measurements represent the thickness of a double layer of skin and the underlying subcutaneous fat. Procedures are simple for obtaining skinfold measurements. It is extremely crucial, however, that the following criteria be adhered to during the measurement: Error within and between investigators can only be minimized when sites are carefully marked and when standard techniques are used for measuring and recording. Individuals performing the procedure must be properly trained in locating the sites and have had sufficient practice to be consistent in measurements. Which skinfold sites to be selected will be based on the purpose of the measurement and the prediction equation selected. The skinfold caliper selected should exert a standard pressure per unit of $10g/mm^2$, such as Lange, Harpenden and Holtain calipers. Low-cost plastic calipers should be avoided, and measurements should never be estimated from a ruler.

A tape measure will be necessary for the skinfolds that require midpoint sites between two landmarks. All skinfold sites should be marked with an erasable pin or marker. The double fold of skin is lifted approximately 1 cm above the mark by placing the thumb and index finger of the left hand roughly 8 cm apart. The two fingers are drawn together to grasp the fold firmly until the measurement is taken. Each arm of the skinfold caliper is placed against the skin so that the jaws of the caliper are perpendicular to the fold. Take the skinfold measurements while the person is standing.

The skinfold will depress with time; therefore, the measurements are usually taken immediately after placing the calipers on the skinfolds. Three measurements should be taken at each site consecutively, never sequentially. Repeat the measurement at each site. Regrasp the skinfold and apply the calipers. Record. If the difference between the two measurements is greater than 0.5 millimeters, take another measurement. Take the average of the three closest readings and use it for the calculations. Ideally, another person should record the measurements during the assessment to avoid bias by the person taking the skinfolds. In the United States measurements are usually performed on the right side, whereas in Europe the left side is selected. Use Tables 7.2 and 7.3 to find the percent body fat.

Table 7.2. How to measure skinfolds. (Illustrations courtesy of N.D.C.)

On males, measure the skinfolds at the subscapula and the right thigh.

Subscapula — the bottom point of the scapula (shoulder blade)

Thigh — the middle of the front side of the thigh halfway between the hip and the knee

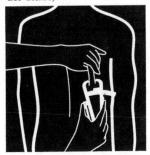 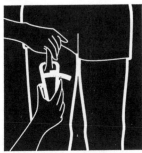

Females are measured at the triceps and the suprailiac sites.

Triceps — the back of the upper arm halfway between the shoulder and the elbow

Suprailiac — just over the top of the hip bone at the middle of the side of the body

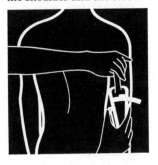 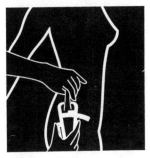

Table 7.3. Conversion of skinfolds to percent body fat.

PERCENT BODY FAT/MEN

PERCENT BODY FAT/WOMEN

SUBSCAPULAR SKINFOLD (MM) — THIGH SKINFOLD (MM) — PERCENT FAT

TRICEPS SKINFOLD (MM) — PERCENT FAT — SUPRAILIAC SKINFOLD (MM)

Source: A.W. Sloan. Estimates of body fat in young men. Journal of Applied Physiology 23:311, 1967.

Source: A.W. Sloan et. al. Estimation of body fat in young women. Journal of Applied Physiology 17:967, 1962.

Since children have different composition of lean muscle mass than adults, the establishment of skinfold equations has been recently established in children. Equations were provided for predicting body fat in children aged 8 to 18 years from triceps and calf skinfolds (in millimeters):

$$\text{boys: } \% \text{ fat} = 0.735 \text{ (triceps} + \text{calf)} + 1.0$$
$$\text{girls: } \% \text{ fat} = 0.610 \text{ (triceps} + \text{calf)} + 5.1$$

Bioelectrical Impedance

The bioelectrical impedance method is based on the conductance of a low amperage electrical current in the body. The method is based on the fact that lean body tissue has a greater amount of water and electrolytes than adipose or fat tissue; therefore, lean body tissue is a good conductor of electricity. This method is essentially a measure of total body water, which is used to estimate lean body mass. Fat weight is then calculated by subtracting lean body weight from body weight. Bioelectrical impedance is popular for mass screening and is an easy and noninvasive technique. Measurements should be made at least 2 hours after consumption of food and within 30 minutes of voiding. Subjects fully clothed, but without socks and shoes, lie on a table with arms away from the body and legs apart. A total of four electrodes are positioned on the dorsal side of the hands and feet.

There are some problems and assumptions associated with bioelectrical impedance. It carries all the problems and errors of formulating a body composition method from the narrow approach of a two-component system. Percentage body fat of lean individuals tends to be overestimated and in obese individuals is underestimated. Dehydration through dieting and the effect of fluid shifts and menstrual cycle on validation of the bioelectrical impedance technique remains unknown.

Optimal Body Composition

For general health, the target percentage of body fat for men is 15 percent; a desirable level of body fat for women is 22 percent. Three percent of the total body fat in men is considered "essential body fat." It appears that man cannot reduce his body fat below this limit without impairing his physiological function and capacity for exercise. The percentage of body fat considered "essential" for women is 12 percent. Women carry more body fat than men for child-bearing functions and the sex specific fat found in the breasts and other tissues. These numbers used to define "essential fat" should **NEVER** be viewed as optimal. A specific percentage fat should not be recommended but rather a range of fatness that is realistic and appropriate for the individual.

A major misuse of optimal body weight prescription is occurring in athletes, especially female athletes. Body weight can be related to performance. There is a point when an athlete can weigh too much, so that performance will be compromised. There is also a point at which the athlete's weight can be too low, and performance declines. Some athletes and coaches believe that the leaner they are, the faster and swifter they will become. Unfortunately, making an athlete leaner than their best competition weight will not allow them to perform better. As a matter of fact, they usually have a decrement in performance. Unhealthy percentages of body fat and total body weights are being established for the female athlete, especially those who participate in lean profile sports such as gymnastics, cross-country running, diving, and figure skating. It is not unusual to hear coaches encourage or request their female athletes to have a percentage body fat lower than 15 percent or telling them that less than 10% is a sign of commitment. Some coaches and athletes have even gone so far as to recommend liposuction surgery to reduce their body fat in certain areas of their bodies, so that they may be more aerodynamic. This obsession to reduce body weight may result in eating disorders among athletes.

Tables are available that compile percentage of body fat for various sports (Table 7.4). These values should never be viewed as the

Table 7.4. Body composition of selected athletes.

Sport	Sex	Age Range	Range of Average % Body Fat
Baseball	M	20-28	11.8-16.2
Outfielders	M	28	9.9
Basketball	F	19-20	20.8-26.9
	M	25-27	7.1-10.6
Bicycling	M	—	8.8
	F		15.4
Football	M	19.3-20.3	13.7-13.9
Defensive backs	M	17-24.5	9.6-11.5
Offensive backs	M	17-24.7	9.4-12.4
Linebackers	M	17-24.7	13.4-14
Lineman	M	17-24.7	15.6-19.1
Quarterbacks	M	24.1	14.4
Hockey	M	22.5-26.3	13.0-15.1
Rowing	M	25.6	6.5

Table 7.4. (*Continued*)

Sport	Sex	Age Range	Range of Average % Body Fat
Racquetball	M	21.0-25.0	8.1-8.5
	F	23	14.0
Speed Skating	M	21.0	9.0-11.4
Figure Skating	M	21.3	9.1
	F	16.5	12.5
Skiing			
Alpine	M	16.5-21.8	9.9-11.0
	F	19.5	20.6
Cross Country	M	21.2-25.6	7.9-12.5
	F	20.2-24.3	15.7-21.8
Nordic	M	21.7	8.9
Soccer			
US Junior	M	17.5	9.4
US Olympic	M	20.6	9.1
US Collegiate	M	20.0	10.9
US National	M	22.5	9.9
Swimming	M	15.1-21.8	5.0-10.8
	F	19.4	26.3
Sprint	F		14.6
Middle Distance	F		24.1
Distance	F		17.1
Synchronized Swimming	F	20.1	24.0
Tennis	M	42	15.2-16.3
	F	39.0	20.3
Track and Field			
Distance Runners	M	22.5-26.2	6.3-4.7
	F	19.9-43.8	15.2-19.2
Middle Distance	M	20.1-24.6	6.9-12.4
Sprint	M	20.1-46.5	5.4-16.5
	F	20.1	19.3
Cross Country	F	15.6	15.3
Race Walking	M	26.7	7.8
Discus	M	26.4-28.3	16.3-16.4
	F	21.1	25.0
Jumper and Hurdlers	F	20.3	20.7
Shot Put	M	22.0-27.0	16.5-19.6
	F	21.5	28.0
Triathlon	M		7.1
	F		12.6
Volleyball	M	26.1	12.0
	F	19.4-21.6	17.9-21.3

Table 7.4. (*Continued*)

Sport	Sex	Age Range	Range of Average % Body Fat
Weight Lifting			
Power	M	24.9-26.3	9.8-19.9
Olympic	M	25.3	12.2
Body Builders	M	25.6-29.0	8.3-13.4
	F	27.0	13.2
Wrestling	M	11.3-27.0	4.0-14.3

Remember these are only estimates of athletes studied. These values should never be viewed as the ideal percentage body fat for an individual athlete. The relative fat percentages cited are the average of the sample selected, NOT the specific percentage for the sport. A specific percentage body fat should not be recommended but rather a range of fatness that is realistic and appropriate for the individual should be used.

Adapted from Wilmore and Costill (1988). *Training for Sport and Activity: The Physiological Basis of the Conditioning Process, 3rd ed.* Dubuque, Iowa: Wm. C. Brown Publishers.

ideal percentage body fat for an individual athlete. The percentages depicted in the table are averages of the athletes measured, not the specific percentage for that sport. Too often the lowest average is viewed as the optimal percentage for maximizing performance. If weight loss is recommended, athletes and coaches need to be educated as to the proper technique to lose the excess fat weight.

PROPER WEIGHT LOSS TECHNIQUES

Athletes should consume at least 1,500-2,000 calories per day to meet nutritional needs as well as their energy needs for training. The daily caloric deficit can range from 500-1,000 calories (depending on the athlete's caloric requirement) not to exceed a two-pound weight loss per week.

This mild caloric restriction results in a manageable loss of water, electrolytes, minerals, and lean body mass and is less likely to cause malnutrition. The weight loss regimen should include 20-30 minutes of aerobic exercise at least three times per week. Some athletes who want to lose weight but don't expend many calories practicing or participating in their sport (gymnastics, figure skating, baseball, and diving) can benefit by adding an aerobic exercise program to increase their caloric expenditure.

Weight loss is most successful when diet and exercise are combined together to create a calorie deficit that results in weight that stays off. Caloric intake can be decreased by eating fewer calories from foods that are calorie dense, such as foods that contain high amounts of sugar, fat and alcohol. Eating habits can also be improved by eating regular meals. Athletes who eat two or three large meals a day will have more difficulty losing weight than do individuals who eat the same amount of calories in five or six meals throughout the day. Also eating smaller more frequent meals spreads the energy intake evenly throughout the day, making energy readily available for training.

Why Not Crash Diet?

Athletes often search for a quick way to lose weight. Fad diets are popular because they promote rapid, temporary weight loss. When crash diets are used to lose weight, the athlete loses lean muscle mass, liver and muscle glycogen, and water, not excess body fat. As a result, athletes fatigue early in their workout or competition, have a hard time keeping training paces, and complain about being tired all the time. Most athletes and coaches regard this rapid weight loss as evidence that they are losing fat, when in fact their body fat stores are virtually untouched.

Long-term problems associated with crash diets include electrolyte imbalances caused by dehydration, iron deficiency anemia, calcium deficiency which may result in decreased bone density, potassium deficiency, weakness, nausea, ketosis and possible kidney problems. Because an athlete's performance will be impaired by the glycogen depletion and resulting dehydration from such a severely restricted diet, fad diets and very low calorie diets used to lose weight are unsuitable for athletes.

Weight Loss Meal Plans

The meal plans found in Table 7.5 are weekly plans for male and female athletes who want to lose weight. These diets emphasize high-carbohydrate, low-fat foods and are based on USDA's Food Guide Pyramid.

For athletes to lose weight safely and effectively, it is important that they eat a variety of foods from each of the five food groups, consume enough carbohydrates to fuel their workouts and lower fat consumption for calorie restriction, rather than following a restrictive fad diet. Table 7.6 lists weight loss guidelines for athletes.

Chronic dieting and repeated weight loss and weight gain (yo-yo dieting) may increase the energy efficiency of the body. This means

Table 7.5.   Meal plans for athletes who plan to lose weight.

The following 2000 calorie diet is an example of a weight loss diet for a **female** athlete who wants to lose weight.

	Carbohydrate (gm)	Calories
BREAKFAST:		
Orange juice, 6 oz.	19	80
Raisin Bran, large bowl	60	240
Skim milk, 1 cup	12	86
Banana	27	105
Total Calories: 511		
Percent Carbohydrate: 92%		
LUNCH:		
Vegetable soup, 1 cup	9	60
Chicken, 2 oz.	0	77
Bagel	31	163
Applesauce, 1 cup	28	100
Low-fat fruited yogurt, 1 cup	42	225
Total Calories: 625		
Percent Carbohydrate: 70%		
DINNER:		
Spaghetti, cooked, 1 cup	37	200
Spaghetti sauce, ⅔ cup	17	114
Broccoli, 1 cup	9	50
Whole wheat roll	15	72
Margarine, 1 pat	0	100
Skim milk, 1 cup	12	86
Total Calories: 622		
Percent Carbohydrate: 57%		
SNACK:		
Mozzarella cheese, 1 oz.	1	80
Pear	25	98
Total Calories: 178		
Percent Carbohydrate: 58%		

The following 3000 calorie diet is an example of a weight loss diet for a **male** athlete who wants to lose weight.

	Carbohydrate (gm)	Calories
BREAKFAST:		
Quaker Oatmeal, apples & cinnamon, 1½ cups	52	268
Whole wheat toast, 2 slices	23	122
Jam or jelly, 2 tsp.	10	36
Margarine, 2 tsp.	0	67

Table 7.5. (*Continued*)

	Carbohydrate (gm)	Calories
Skim milk, 1 cup	12	86
Orange juice, 8 oz.	27	112

Total Calories: 691
Percent Carbohydrate: 71%

LUNCH:

	Carbohydrate (gm)	Calories
Ham sandwich		
2 oz. ham	1	97
1 slice tomato	1	5
1 tsp. mustard	trace	4
1 tsp. mayonnaise	1	19
lettuce		
2 slices whole wheat bread	26	140
Skim milk, 1 cup	12	86
Banana	27	105
Blueberry muffin	20	126
Tomato soup, 2 cups	44	320

Total Calories: 902
Percent Carbohydrate: 58%

DINNER:

	Carbohydrate (gm)	Calories
Flank steak, broiled, 3 oz.	0	243
Large baked potato	51	220
Margarine, 2 tsp.	0	67
Peas, 1 cup	25	134
Carrot sticks, 1 cup	15	62
Skim milk, 1 cup	12	86
Apple	21	81

Total Calories: 893
Percent Carbohydrate: 55%

MID-MORNING SNACK:

	Carbohydrate (gm)	Calories
Low-fat fruited yogurt, 1 cup	42	225
Bagel	31	163
Peanut butter, 2 tsp.	2	63

AFTERNOON SNACK:

	Carbohydrate (gm)	Calories
Pear	25	98
Grapefruit juice, 1 cup	24	102

Total Calories: 651
Percent Carbohydrate: 76%

Table 7.6. Weight loss guidelines.

- Goal: to lose 1-2 pounds per week
- Reduce calories by 500-1,000 per day
    **never drop below 1,200 calories per day
- Reduce fats, high-calorie and low-nutrient density foods like chips and nuts
- Engage in aerobic exercise for at least 30-40 minutes 3 times per week
- Don't try to lose weight during the season or during peak performance times
- Add an aerobic activity if you are involved in a low-intensity sport like baseball or gymnastics.

the body adapts to fewer calories. For example, after repeated yo-yo dieting an individual who was able to lose weight on a 1,500 calorie diet in the past, may no longer lose weight eating 1,500 calories. To lose weight, they have to drop the calorie level even lower. The resistance to weight loss in yo-yo dieting, as with fad dieting, is thought to occur due to a decreased metabolic rate. The body may respond to these extremely low-calorie diets by lowering its metabolic rate to defend what it perceives as starvation. Although there is controversy to whether or not yo-yo dieting lowers metabolic rate it may alter body composition, specifically increasing the proportion of fat to lean tissue.

Eating Disorders

Concern about harmful methods of weight control and patterns of disordered eating is increasing in the athletic world. These methods range from the use of diet pills, laxatives, and diuretics to fasting, severe dieting, binging, and self-induced vomiting. Although these practices themselves do not confirm that an eating disorder exists, they may place the athlete at an increased risk for developing a more serious problem.

Several researchers have reported that among female collegiate athletes, 32 percent practice at least one pathogenic weight-control behavior daily. Pathogenic weight-control behaviors were defined as self-induced vomiting or the abuse of laxatives, diet pills, or diuretics. Those athletes that participate in lean profile sports such as distance running, gymnastics, figure skating, swimming, wrestling, and judo may be especially vulnerable. A survey of 42 female college gymnasts showed that all were dieting and that 26 (62%) were using at least one pathogenic weight-control technique. In addition, 21 of the 28 competitors (75%), who were told by their coaches they were too heavy, resorted to using pathogenic weight-control behaviors. A survey of 9 to

18-year-old swimmers reported that 15 percent of the girls and 4 percent of the boys used pathogenic weight-loss methods. Some of the swimmers began using these behaviors at a young age: 9 years (dieting), 10 years (fasting), 11 years (self-induced vomiting), 12 years (diuretics), and 14 years (laxatives). Extreme dieting and distortions in body image have been also reported in male athletes and appear to be increasing in number the last few years. Athletes in sports that do not focus on weight, such as basketball, hockey, and volleyball may be at a lower risk of developing eating disorders.

Symptomatology

Because eating disorders can have serious medical consequences, it is extremely important for athletes to seek prompt medical and psychologic attention if symptoms of anorexia or bulimia are detected. In fact, early treatment of eating disorders is the number one factor of a successful recovery. Treatment usually involves a multidisciplinary approach that includes medical care, psychology and nutrition counseling.

Anorexia Nervosa

Anorexia nervosa is characterized by an intense fear of becoming overweight which leads the individual to a persistent, intentional weight loss, and maintenance of weight at a very low, unhealthy level. Anorexics also do not have an accurate perception of their own bodies. They see themselves as being fat even if they are underweight. These abnormal perceptions are often based on feelings of powerlessness, lack of control and poor self-esteem.

The diagnostic criteria for anorexia nervosa are found in Table 7.7.

Table 7.7. Diagnostic criteria for anorexia nervosa.

- Refusal to maintain body weight over minimal normal weight for age and height (e.g., weight loss leading to maintenance of body weight 15 percent below what is expected) or failure to make expected weight gain during period of growth, leading to body weight 15 percent below what is expected.
- Intense fear of weight gain or becoming fat, even though underweight.
- Disturbance in the way in which one's body weight, size, or shape is experienced (e.g., the person claims to "feel fat" even when emaciated; believes that one area of the body is "too fat" even when obviously underweight).
- In females, absence of at least three consecutive menstrual cycles when otherwise expected to occur (primary or secondary amenorrhea). A woman is considered to have amenorrhea if her periods occur only following hormone adminstration (e.g., estrogen).

From: *Diagnostic and Statistical Manual of Mental Disorders*, ed. by the American Psychiatric Association, 1987.

Bulimia Nervosa

Bulimia is characterized by a binge-purge syndrome that involves the consumption of large amounts of food that are high in calories followed by purging (self-induced vomiting, laxative or diuretic abuse). Binging, which may be triggered by a stressful situation or a period of restrictive eating such as a fad diet, serves as a way of coping with the environment. The individual then seeks relief from the physical distress and emotional pain and guilt by purging. Bulimics are also overly concerned with body weight. However, unlike the anorexics, bulimics are usually of normal weight or above normal weight. The diagnostic criteria for bulimia nervosa is listed in Table 7.8.

Table 7.8. Diagnostic criteria for bulimia nervosa.

- Recurrent episodes of binge eating (rapid consumption of large amounts of food in discrete period of time).
- A feeling of lack of control over eating behavior during the eating binges.
- The person regularly engages in either self-induced vomiting, use of laxatives or diuretics, strict dieting or fasting, or vigorous exercise in order to prevent weight gain.
- A minimum average of two binge-eating episodes a week for at least 3 months.
- Persistant over-concern with body shape and weight.

From: *Diagnostic and Statistical Manual of Mental Disorders*, ed. by the American Psychiatric Association, 1987.

Many of these behaviors do not, by themselves, prove the presence of an eating disorder, but identification of one or more may justify further attention to the possible presence of a problem.

Common complaints of eating disorders include fatigue (or denial of fatigue when it would be appropriate), dizziness, persistent chills, abdominal discomfort with constipation or diarrhea, amenorrhea, stress fractures, shin splints, and insomnia. Psychologic symptoms include increased anxiety or agitation, bizarre preoccupation with food, excessive pride in weight loss combined with a denial of thinness, loss of pleasure in activities usually enjoyed, withdrawal from people and social interactions, and feelings of hopelessness and despair.

Anorectics and athletes have similar characteristics; diagnosis of an eating disorder in athletes is often a challenge. Shared and distinguishing traits of the weight-preoccupied athlete and the patient with anorexia are listed in Table 7.9.

Athletes suspected of having an eating disorder need professional help. These athletes should be approached privately, by someone they trust and assured that confidentiality will be maintained. It is possible that the eating disordered athlete may not accept any offer for help. Ultimately, it is the athlete who must make the first step toward treat-

Table 7.9. Characteristics of anorectic and athletic women.

| SHARED FEATURES | DISTINGUISHING FEATURES | |
	Athlete	Anorectic
Dietary faddism	Purposeful training	Aimless physical activity
Controlled calorie consumption	Increased exercise tolerance	Poor or decreasing exercise performance
Specific carbohydrate avoidance	Good muscle development, accurate body image	Poor muscle development, flawed body image (always over weight)
Low body weight	Body fat level within defined range	Body fat level below normal range
Slow pulse and low blood pressure		Biochemical abnormalities if abusing laxatives or diuretics
Increased physical activity		
Amenorrhea or Oligomenorrhea		
Anemia (may or may not be present)		

Source: Reprinted from *American Family Physician*, American Academy of Family Physicians February 1984.

ment and recovery, however, if they have been confronted with the knowledge of their eating disorder, at least they will have someone to turn to for help in the future.

Complications

Many serious complications are associated with eating disorders; if allowed to persist many can be life-threatening as in the case of the Olympic gymnast who died due to complications of anorexia nervosa in 1994. Medical complications associated with anorexia and/or bulimia are listed in Table 7.10. Recent evidence that anorexia, men-

Table 7.10. Medical characteristics of eating disorders for anorexia and bulimia.

- Menstrual irregularities and/or amenorrhea
- Dental and gum disease
- Swollen partoid glands
- Gastrointestinal problems
- Electrolyte abnormalities and dehydration
- Cardiac arrhythmias
- Hypotension

strual dysfunction (athletic amenorrhea) and bone mineral disorders (reduced bone mineral density) form a triad of disorders in certain female athletes. It appears that the female athlete can enter any one of these practices and be suspect to an underlying eating disorder.

Prevention

No one can guarantee that an eating disorder will not happen, however, prevention can be best accomplished when coaches, parents and athletes sit down and candidly discuss the risks of eating disorders among themselves. Athletes, particularly young female and male athletes, need to learn how to lose weight the correct and safe way, rather than choosing restricted calorie diets or fad diets. Ninety percent of eating disorders stem from an athlete having success at losing weight on a fad diet.

If a serious disorder is detected, the athlete should not compete until treatment is started. If the disorder remains untreated, the athlete may suffer permanent physical injury. Table 7.11 lists organizations

Table 7.11. Resources for individuals with eating disorders as well as for their families and health care professionals.

American Anorexia/Bulimia Association, Inc.
418 East 76th Street
New York, NY 10021
(212) 734-1114

Anorexia Nervosa and Related Eating Disorders (ANRED)
P.O. Box 5102
Eugene, OR 97405
(503) 344-1144

National Anorexic Aid Society (NAAS)
5796 Karl Road
Columbus, OH 43229
(614) 436-1112

National Association of Anorexia and Associated Disorders (ANAD)
P.O. Box 271
Highland Park, IL 60035
(708) 831-3438

National Collegiate Athletic Association (NCAA)
Video Tapes on Eating Disorders
Karol Media
350 N. Pennsylvania Ave.
Box 7600
Wilkes-Barre, PA 18773-7600
1-800-526-4773

that will disseminate information and help for individuals with an eating disorder.

WEIGHT GAIN

During a Taper or Off Season

Kim is your best swimmer on the team. She performed well at the Nationals and now has the next 4 weeks off. You tell her to take it easy and relax during the break. A month later she shows up at the pool 7 pounds heavier and claiming she watched her calorie intake over the break.

There are some physiological changes in the body that occur during detraining that could explain why athletes tend to gain weight during their break or even taper, other than just eating too much food.

Some of the research investigating weight gain has focused on an enzyme called Lipoprotein Lipase (LPL). Both fat cells and muscle cells produce LPL to help them store energy as fat. The LPL enzyme at the cells captures the circulating fat after a meal and stores it either in muscles, where it is used as a fuel for exercise, or fat, where it is stored. As you might expect, obese people have much more LPL activity in their fat cells than lean athletes. The activity of LPL is also influenced by weight loss. A group of researchers found that LPL activity rose after weight loss and may serve as a signal to the gene that produces the LPL enzyme, saying "make more enzyme to store fat." This response to weight loss may explain why lost weight is so easily regained.

Recently, Simsolo and colleagues reported on new research in the area of LPL and exercise in the *Journal of Clinical Investigations* (92:2124-2130, 1993). Their study examined the effects of exercise on LPL activity and indicated that during training or regular consistent exercise, LPL activity at the muscle is higher than at the fat cell. However, with detraining, such as a break at the end of the swimming season, LPL activity is higher at the fat cell than at the muscle. This increase in fat cell LPL coupled with a decrease in muscle LPL yields a condition favoring fat tissue storage. Thus, detraining of athletes may result in heavier weights and increased body fat percentages.

To prevent weight gain or increased fat stores during the end of the season break, or during a taper, athletes should be advised to continue some type of fitness regimen or physical activity program to keep the LPL activity in the skeletal muscles active. For example, Kim doesn't need to keep on swimming, but a regular consistent physical fitness program and a sensible diet low in fat should be helpful.

Weight Gain for Muscular Strength and Endurance

When it comes to weight, most sports active individuals are content to maintain their desired weight, while others wish they could gain weight. Usually hockey, football and basketball players, body builders, and teenage boys want to gain weight by building muscles. In order to gain weight, athletes need to consume more calories than they expend in workouts and daily living. This sounds simple, but may not be since it takes longer to gain weight than to lose it.

Family history plays a major role in the natural development of an athlete's physique. Athletes from naturally thin families are less likely to be able to transform their bodies from thin svelte figures to bulky muscular ones. With improved nutrition and appropriate weight training, however, athletes can enhance their likelihood of gaining weight. With age, many young athletes will naturally gain weight.

Keys to Gaining Weight

Dereck, a young redshirted freshman, was 6'8" and weighed 250 pounds. He had been told to gain between 20-30 pounds during his freshman year in order to get the starting position for the team next year. He had been eating everything in site and was tired of overeating. He resorted to consuming foods that were very high in calories in order to cut down on the amount of foods he had to consume. As a result he started to consume about a quart of half-and-half a day. Dereck found the half-and-half easy to drink and store in his dorm room refrigerator. It was high in calories and provided the extra calories that he needed in order to gain weight. The problem was that he was consuming nothing but pure fat. While he had no family history of heart disease, there is no better way to start a young man on the road to coronary heart disease than drinking a quart of half-and-half on a daily basis. He was putting diesel gasoline in a tank that needed super unleaded gasoline. He needed to stop drinking the half-and-half and take in about 500-1000 extra calories per day, mostly in the form of carbohydrates with some extra protein.

Some examples of the foods Dereck needed were a peanut butter sandwich with a glass of milk as a snack before bed; a banana instead of an apple for more calories; cranberry, apple and grape juices instead of orange juice; instant breakfast drinks as snacks or a supplement during the day or in the mornings when he had an early class and skipped breakfast.

Although it took him almost 2 years to successfully add 30 pounds of lean muscle mass, Dereck became a starter on the varsity football team and has been touted as one of the best collegiate offensive linemen in the country with potential NFL skills.

Muscle can be gained through intense strength training several times a week coupled with the consumption of additional calories. For each pound gained as muscle, the athlete will need to consume about 500-1000 extra calories per day. The extra calories should come from a variety of foods, milk, meat, fruits, vegetables, and grains. Consistency is the key. Eating three meals a day with snacks in between is an essential key to gaining lean body mass. Athletes who sleep in and skip breakfast miss an opportunity to add carbohydrate calories to their diet. When eating, athletes should eat enough to satisfy their appetite and then eat a little more. This can be accomplished by: eating larger than normal portions, eating an extra snack or additional meal (like a peanut butter sandwich with milk), drinking commercial or homemade liquid meals with regular meals or as snacks. Bulky, low-calorie foods, such as cereal, grain, and salads should be held to a minimum as they are too filling in relationship to the amount of calories they provide. Table 7.12 provides sample menu patterns for healthy, high-calorie, carbohydrate-rich meals.

Table 7.12. Sample 5000-6000 calorie diets.

Sample 1

Breakfast

1 cup orange juice
1 cup oatmeal
1 cup 2% milk
1 scrambled egg
2 slices of toast
Jam or jelly

Snacks

1 peanut butter sandwich
1 banana
1 cup juice

Lunch

1 large cheeseburger
1 large serving french fries
Tossed salad with dressing
1 cup 2% milk
1 piece cake or pie or cookies
Fresh fruit (apple, orange, banana)

Snacks

2 ounces of cheese
10 crackers
1 cup yogurt

Dinner

1 cup soup
4 ounces chicken (2 chicken breasts)
1 cup sweet potatoes or 1½ cups rice
2 dinner rolls or bread
1 cup vegetables
Tossed salad with dressing or coleslaw
Fresh fruit or fruit juice
1 cup 2% milk

Snacks

Milkshake or ice cream
Hot chocolate with cookie

Table 7.12. (*Continued*)

Sample 2

Breakfast
1½ cups cold cereal
2 cups 2% milk
1 banana
2 cups orange juice
2 slices of whole wheat toast
or English muffin
Jam or jelly

Snacks
Package of raisins with fruit juice
  or 2% milk
Bagel with peanut butter

Lunch
2 slices whole wheat bread
2 Tbsp. peanut butter
Apple
Low-fat yogurt
Tossed salad with dressing
1 cup 2% milk
Carrot sticks

Snacks
2 ounces of cheese
10 crackers
Fresh fruit
1 cup 2% milk

Dinner
4 ounces of chicken (2 chicken breasts)
1 large baked potato with 2 pats butter
1 cup mixed vegetables
2 slices whole wheat bread
Tossed salad with dressing
1 cup ice cream
1 cup 2% milk

Snacks
Brownie with milk
popcorn

Sample 3

Breakfast
2 waffles, or pancakes with syrup
1 scrambled egg
1 cup orange juice
1 cup 2% milk

Snacks
Yogurt
Banana with peanut butter

Lunch
4 ounces roast beef
2 cups mashed potatoes (gravy if desired)
1 cup of vegetables
2 slices of bread
Fresh fruit or fruit juice
Cake, pie or cookies
1 cup 2% milk

Snacks
Milkshake or ice cream
Package of nuts
Fruit juice

Dinner
3 cups spaghetti with meat sauce
Tossed salad with dressing
2 slices garlic bread
1 cup 2% milk
Ice cream with fruit sauce (i.e., strawberries,
  or a banana or peaches, cut up)

Snacks
Apple w/2 ounces cheese
Cold cereal with milk

8 Eating On The Road

"One of the nice things about the Senior Tour is we can take a cart and cooler. If your game is not going well, you can always have a picnic."
—*Lee Trevino*

INTRODUCTION

Competing on the road presents a number of challenges for athletes. Jet lag, unfamiliar playing fields and sites, changes in sleep and training are just a few of the obstacles you and your teammates face. No matter where you are competing, it is important to chose the right fuel for optimal performance. Too often traveling athletes will skip meals, eat insufficient amounts of carbohydrates, and compete dehydrated. Athletes who consume diets that are chronically deficient in carbohydrates and fluid can experience a progressive depletion of glycogen stores which may cause a drop in endurance, precision, and speed.

MAKING WISE FOOD CHOICES

The first rule to making wise food choices on the road is to determine where you will eat before mealtime arrives. Simply put, PLAN AHEAD. Try to find a suitable restaurant and ask for a pasta meal within your budget. Usually, the manager or chef can accommodate you, especially if you make this request on a regular basis. Pasta meals, burritos with beans and rice, cold cereal with low-fat milk, baked potatoes, and fruits and vegetables can usually be found in restaurants and provide the easiest and cheapest sources of carbohydrates (see Table 8.1).

If you stay in a hotel that offers food service, contact the catering manager and request high-carbohydrate meals within your budget.

Remember, as long as you are paying for the meals, you can usually demand the type and quality of food desired. Don't be afraid to ask for special foods, and make sure you get a reasonable price. The hotel or restaurant wants your business. Ordering *a la carte* might be

Table 8.1. Guidelines for choosing meals while traveling.

BREAKFAST HINTS

- Try pancakes, waffles, french toast, bagels, muffins, cereal, fruit or juices for a high-carbohydrate breakfast.
- Juice, dried fruit, fresh fruit, pretzels and bagels are good snacks to pack when away from home.
- Breakfast is the easiest meal to consume carbohydrate-rich foods.
- Avoid meals that contain high-fat choices such as bacon or sausage.

Suggested Breakfast Menus:

Orange juice, 1 cup Pancakes with syrup (3) 1 banana sliced on pancakes	547 calories, 90% carbohydrate
Apple juice, 6 ounces Raisin Bran, large bowl Low-fat milk, 1 cup Banana	498 calories, 95% carbohydrate
Bran muffin, large Hot cocoa Raisins or fresh fruit	310 calories, 69% carbohydrate
Plain English muffin, 1 Strawberry jam, 2 T. Scrambled egg, 1 Orange juice, 1 cup Low-fat yogurt, 1 cup	580 calories, 69% carbohydrates

LUNCH HINTS

- Emphasize the bread in sandwiches rather than the fillings.
- Avoid double hamburgers with cheese and bacon, fried fish, fried chicken and french fries at fast food restaurants.
- Try baked potatoes, salads with fat-free dressing, plain hamburgers, chili or plain burritos and tacos at fast food restaurants as they have less fat.
- Choose fruit juices or low-fat milk rather than soft drinks.

Suggested Lunch Menus:

Large turkey sandwich on two slices of bread Low-fat fruited yogurt, 1 cup Orange juice, 1 cup	1017 calories, 60% carbohydrate
Plain baked potato Chili, 1 cup Chocolate milkshake	916 calories, 62% carbohydrate
Vegetable soup, 1 cup Baked chicken, 1 breast Bread, 1 slice Applesauce, 1 cup Low-fat fruited yogurt, 1 cup	737 calories, 71% carbohydrate

Table 8.1. (*Continued*)

DINNER HINTS

- When on the road find a restaurant that offers pasta, baked potatoes, rice, breads, vegetables and salads.
- Order thick crust pizza and double the amount of vegetable toppings like green peppers, mushrooms, onions, tomatoes, instead of pepperoni and sausage.
- Try restaurants that offer Italian foods such as spaghetti, lasagna, breads and salads.
- Vegetable soups accompanied by crackers, bread, and muffins can add to a low-fat, carbohydrate-rich meal.

Suggested Dinner Menus:

Minestrone soup, 1 cup
Spaghetti, 2 cups
Marinara sauce, ⅔ cup
Parmesan cheese, 1 T.
Breadsticks, 2
Low-fat milk, 1 cup   977 calories, 68% carbohydrates

Turkey, 4 ounces
Stuffing, ½ cup
Mashed potatoes, 1 cup
Peas, 1 cup
Roll, 1
Low-fat milk, 1 cup   960 calories, 55% carbohydrate

Lean roast beef, 3 ounces
Rice, 1½ cup
Corn, 1 cup
Rolls, 2
Low-fat milk, 1½ cup   1320 calories, 60% carbohydrates

---

more expensive but it has its advantages of offering greater variety and can increase the carbohydrate content of your diet.

In many restaurants if you speak up and are polite, you can request substitutions. Request a baked potato instead of french fries, whole wheat bread for white bread, jelly instead of fat-loaded pats of butter, skim milk or fruit juice instead of calorie-dense soda pop, and ask for your salad dressing on the side to help control the amount of fat in your diet.

Approach buffets with caution. It is tempting to regard buffet dining as a personal challenge, with the goal to get more than your money's worth by filling up your plate till it is overflowing. Instead, survey the entire buffet line, decide what foods are high in carbohydrate and low in fat, and stick to those foods. Fill up on nutritious foods first and that way you will get all the fuel and nutrients you need to compete and stay healthy.

When making food selections at restaurants, athletes and coaches should also pay careful attention to key words when making menu selections for increasing carbohydrates and lowering fat consumption (see Table 8.2).

Table 8.2. Key words to look for when reading a menu.

1. Fat content must be watched when selecting menu items. If you see one of the following words describing a food, try to make another selection: **FRIED, CRISPY, BREADED, SCAMPI STYLE, CREAMED, BUTTERY, AU GRATIN, GRAVY.**
2. Selection adjectives that are good and represent lower fat foods are: **MARINARA, STEAMED, BOILED, BROILED, TOMATO SAUCE, IN ITS OWN JUICE, POACHED, CHARBROILED.**
3. Restaurant Choices. Depending on the restaurant you go to, here are some tips when selecting foods:
   - **MEXICAN** Choose low-fat refried beans or refried beans with no lard. Try chicken or lean beef and bean burritos. Ask for baked soft corn tortillas instead of deep fat fried shells or flour tortillas. Use salsa instead of sour cream and guacamole. Fill up on rice and flour tortillas. Watch the chip intake.
   - **ITALIAN** Pasta with marinara sauce is good, but watch the cream sauces. Pizza, plain or with vegetables, is a good choice. Salads with dressing on the side and bread with butter on the side are good choices. Low-fat Italian ices and low-fat frozen yogurt are better than rich dessert choices.
   - **CHINESE** Stir fry and steamed dishes, such as chicken and vegetables with rice, are good choices. Minimize your intake of deep fried items such as egg rolls, wontons, and sweet and sour pork.
   - **BURGER PLACES** Salad bars are great, but use a low-fat or nonfat dressing. Look for grilled burgers, hold the mayonnaise and go light on the cheese. Watch your french fry intake (select a baked potato with a topping on the side if you can), and drink juice or low-fat milk instead of the milkshake.
   - **BREAKFAST CAFES** Always ask for margarine on the side when ordering pancakes, toast, bagels and waffles. Select fruit, fruit juices, and whole grain cereals, breads, and muffins. Watch your caffeine intake.

If you can't afford all three meals at a restaurant, choose breakfast. With selections like cereal (hot or cold), bagels, English muffins, pancakes, toast, fruit and fruit juices, breakfast can be inexpensive and an easy way to get carbohydrate-rich foods.

If your budget does not allow restaurant meals or if you only have a day trip, a nearby grocery store offers a great variety of foods. They may have a delicatessen or a soup and salad bar, and you can always pick up fresh fruits, vegetables, fruit juices, low-fat milk and dairy products as well as breads, bagels, muffins and low-fat luncheon meats. Not only are grocery stores easy and fast, they can also be a cheaper source of meals than restaurants. Athletes can choose foods from all five food groups and come away with nutritious food choices that can enhance their performance.

Another way to eat more nutrient-dense foods is to bring or pack nutritious snacks for the road trip. Usually, athletes who travel by bus or van tend to consume candy, soda pop, and potato chips. To cut down on these types of foods, pack a cooler with more nutrient-dense munchies like fresh and dried fruit, Fig Newtons, "energy bars" and cans of fruit juice. Table 8.3 lists examples of nutritious, high-carbohydrate snacks for athletes who are traveling.

Table 8.3. Packing the cooler.

• Fluids — water, sport drinks, fruit juices	• Bagels, breads and rolls
• Turkey sandwiches	• Rice cakes
• Fresh and dried fruit	• Breadsticks
• Low- or non-fat yogurt	• Pretzels
• Vegetables	• Graham crackers
• Part-skim string cheese	• Animal crackers
• Energy bars	• Fig bars, nutrigrain bars
• Low-fat ready-to-eat cereal	• Ginger snaps and vanilla wafers

SMART FOOD CHOICES AT FAST FOOD RESTAURANTS

It's 7:00 p.m. and you've just finished competing. You shower, dress, and pile into the team bus or van. It's now 8:15 p.m. You're starving, on a limited budget, and you have a two-hour drive home. *WHERE DO YOU EAT?* Like many traveling teams and athletes, you stop at a fast food restaurant. Although fast foods can be high in fat and low in calcium and in vitamins A and C, an athlete can make wise food selections by using the charts shown in Tables 8.4 and 8.5.

By making a few wise food choices at fast food restaurants, you can change a calorie-dense meal into a nutrient-dense meal. Next time you step up to the counter to order your fast food feast:

- Think about what you've already eaten and what you'll eat later in the day. Fit this into your food intake for the entire day. For example, if you had a deluxe meal combo, you might decide to cut back and have a lighter dinner.
- Try to include low-fat dairy products and at least two vegetables or fruits with each meal.
- Limit the amount of salad dressing (or use fat-free), mayonnaise, and other special sauces.

Table 8.4. Smart food choices at fast food restaurants.

Meals	Serving	Calories	Protein	CHO	Fat
Breakfast					
McDonald's					
Apple bran muffin	1	650	17%	52%	26%
Breakfast burrito	1				
Orange juice	6 oz.				
1% milk	8 oz.				
Hot cakes with syrup, 2 pats butter	3	660	13%	58%	30%
Scrambled egg					
Orange juice	6 oz.				
Apple bran muffin	1	650	20%	64%	21%
Egg McMuffin	1				
1% milk	8 oz.				
Orange juice	6 oz.				
Burger King					
Bagel	1	475	16%	64%	21%
Jam	1				
2% milk	8 oz.				
Orange juice	6 oz.				
Lunch/Dinner					
McDonald's					
McLean deluxe	1	547	21%	61%	19%
Side salad	1				
Lite Vinaigrette	1 pkt.				
Orange juice	6 oz.				
Vanilla yogurt cone	1				
Wendy's					
Grilled chicken sandwich	1	820	19%	57%	26%
Baked potato	1				
Sour cream	1 pkt.				
Margarine	1 pat				
2% milk	8 oz.				
Jr. hamburger	1	820	12%	66%	25%
Baked potato with broccoli and cheese	1				
Lemonade	8 oz.				
Hardee's					
Grilled chicken sandwich	1	790	14%	57%	22%
Mashed potatoes	4 oz.				
Gravy	1.5 oz.				
Chocolate shake	Medium				
Arby's					
Light roasted chicken deluxe	1	644	21%	57%	24%
Jamoca shake	Medium				

Table 8.4. (*Continued*)

Meals	Serving	Calories	Protein	CHO	Fat
Pizza Hut					
Spaghetti with meat sauce	1 order	1,023	19%	61%	20%
Breadsticks	1 order				
2% or skim milk	8 oz.				
Pizza with onion and green pepper (thin crust-medium)	4 slices	1,126	20%	55%	25%
Breadsticks	1 order				
2% or skim milk	8 oz.				
Subway					
Turkey on whole wheat	6″	850	24%	50%	26%
Side salad	1				
Lite Italian dressing	1 pkt.				
2% or skim milk	8 oz.				

Table 8.5. Fast food.

To determine the percentage of calories from fat in a food, multiply the grams of fat in that food by 9. Then divide that number by the total number of calories in that food.

For example: Food X has 350 calories and 15 grams of fat.

$$\begin{array}{r} 15 \text{ (grams of fat)} \\ \times\ 9 \\ \hline 135 \end{array}$$

$$350 \text{ (total calories)} \overline{\smash{)}135 \text{ (calories from fat)}} = 39\%$$

Therefore, 39 percent of the calories in food X are from fat.

Type of Food	Calories	Protein (gm)	Carbohydrate (gm)	Fat (gm)
Arby's				
Beef and Cheese	459	28	43	26
Club Sandwich	572	31	44	31
Ham and Cheese	355	22	31	16
Roast Beef	347	22	32	15
Super Roast Beef	685	33	67	31
Turkey Deluxe	492	27	44	23
Baked Potato, plain	290	8	66	.5
Potato Cakes (2)	210	2	22	14

Table 8.5. (*Continued*)

Type of Food	Calories	Protein (gm)	Carbohydrate (gm)	Fat (gm)
Burger King				
Ham, Egg Sandwich	335	17	20	20
French Toast Sticks	499	9	49	29
Scrambled Egg Platter	468	15	33	30
Cheeseburger	360	18	35	16
Double Cheeseburger	523	32	35	28
Hamburger	310	16	35	12
Whopper Junior	370	16	35	18
Whopper Junior with Cheese	419	19	35	21
Whopper	669	27	56	38
Whopper with Cheese	761	33	56	45
Chicken Sandwich	685	26	52	42
Chicken Tenders	204	20	10	10
BK Broiler	379	24	31	18
Whaler	540	24	57	24
French Fries, regular	210	3	25	11
Onion Rings	271	3	29	16
Chef Salad	180	17	7	9
Garden Salad	90	6	7	5
Apple Pie	328	3	48	14
Dairy Queen				
Brazier Hamburger	257	13	28	9
Big Brazier, regular	454	27	37	23
Big Brazier, deluxe	470	28	36	24
Brazier Hot Dog	273	11	23	15
Brazier Cheese Dog	225	15	24	19
Brazier Chili Dog	327	13	25	20
Fish Sandwich	401	20	41	17
Onion Rings	301	6	33	17
French Fries, large	315	3	39	16
Ice Cream Cone, medium	227	6	34	7
Buster Ice Cream Bar	389	10	37	22
Mr. Misty, Float	443	6	87	8
Banana Split	535	10	90	15
Ice Cream Sundae, Chocolate	309	6	53	5
Chocolate Malt, large	840	22	125	28
Kentucky Fried Chicken				
Original Recipe, 9 pc	1849	148	58	113
Original Recipe, drumstick	115	12	3	6
Original Recipe, thigh	255	18	6	18
Original Recipe, wing	133	9	4	9
Original Recipe, dinner	846	53	57	47
Extra Crispy, dinner	955	52	63	54
Extra Crispy, 9 pc	2585	150	104	174
Mashed Potatoes	64	2	1	1

Table 8.5. (*Continued*)

Type of Food	Calories	Protein (gm)	Carbohydrate (gm)	Fat (gm)
Gravy	23	0	1	2
Cole Slaw	122	1	13	8
Rolls	61	2	11	1
Biscuit (1)	269	5	32	14
Long John Silver's				
Treasure Chest	506	30	32	33
Fish w/batter (2 pc)	366	22	21	22
Peg Legs w/batter (5 pc)	350	22	26	28
Fish Sandwich	337	22	49	31
Ocean Scallops (6 pc)	283	11	30	13
Shrimp w/batter (6 pc)	268	8	30	13
Seafood Salad	270	16	36	7
Garden Salad	170	9	13	9
French Fries	288	4	33	16
Hush Puppies (3)	153	3	20	7
McDonald's				
Bacon, Egg & Cheese Biscuit	483	16	33	31
Plain Biscuit	330	5	36	18
Egg McMuffin	337	18	31	15
Hamburger	264	12	28	11
Cheeseburger	315	15	28	16
Big Mac	570	25	39	35
McDLT	681	30	40	44
McRib	459	26	43	20
Quarter Pounder w/cheese	525	29	30	32
Chicken McNuggets	323	19	14	21
Filet-O-Fish	432	15	36	26
Chef Salad	230	21	8	13
Garden Salad	110	7	6	7
French Fries	220	3	26	11
Apple Pie	253	2	29	14
Apple Danish	389	6	51	18
Iced Cheese Danish	395	7	42	22
Pizza Hut				
Thin & Crispy Cheese	340	19	32	11
Thin & Crispy Pepperoni	370	19	42	15
Thin & Crispy Pork/Mushroom	450	26	46	19
Thin & Crispy Supreme	400	21	44	17
Thin & Crispy Sup. Supreme	520	30	46	26
Thick & Chewy Cheese	390	24	53	10
Thick & Chewy Pepperoni	450	25	52	16
Thick & Chewy Supreme	480	29	52	18
Thick & Chewy Sup. Supreme	590	34	55	26

(all values for two slices from a medium pizza)

Table 8.5. (*Continued*)

Type of Food	Calories	Protein (gm)	Carbohydrate (gm)	Fat (gm)
Taco Bell				
Bellbeefer w/cheese	278	19	23	12
Bellbeefer	220	15	23	7
Burrito Supreme	452	21	43	22
Bean Burrito	340	11	47	12
Beef Burrito	464	30	37	21
Enchirito	449	25	42	21
Taco	183	15	14	8
Beefy Tostada	289	19	21	15
Combination Burrito	403	21	43	16
Tostada	179	9	25	6
Pintos 'n Cheese	167	11	21	5
Wendy's				
Breakfast Sandwich	369	17	33	19
Omelet, ham/cheese	249	18	6	17
Omelet, ham/cheese/mushroom	288	18	7	21
Omelet, ham/mush/grn pepper	277	19	7	19
Omelet, mush/onion/grn pepper	209	14	7	15
Cheeseburger, double	796	50	41	48
Cheeseburger, single	576	33	34	34
Chicken Sandwich, grain bun	317	25	31	10
Hamburger, double	667	44	34	39
Hamburger, single	472	26	33	26
Chili	228	20	21	8
Garden Salad	102	7	9	5
French Fries	328	5	41	16
Baked Potato w/cheese	599	17	56	35
Baked Potato, chili cheese	510	22	63	20
Baked Potato, plain	250	6	52	2
Frosty	393	9	53	16

- Try some of the new lower fat versions at your favorite fast food chain (like the McLean Deluxe).
- Share fries, a large sandwich, a baked potato, or dessert with a friend. Or take half home for another meal.

INTERNATIONAL TRAVEL

While making wise food choices on the road is no easy task, trying to find familiar and nutritious foods during international travel and competition is extremely difficult. Most athletes who travel internationally have problems finding enough food, as well as finding foods that are familiar and have been prepared in a way that doesn't present any potential food safety hazard.

Problems and Solutions

Athletes who travel to other countries have a 50-50 chance of contracting traveler's diarrhea, a sometimes serious, always annoying, bacterial infection of the digestive tract. The risk is high because other countries' cleanliness standards for food and water are often lower than those of the United States and Canada. In addition, every region's microbes are different, and while people are immune to those in their own neighborhoods, they have not had the chance to develop immunity to the pathogens in the places they are competing.

To protect health against disease-causing organisms not found at home, traveling athletes should drink only bottled water, even if just brushing their teeth. Drink only boiled, bottled, canned or carbonated beverages **without ice cubes.** This way you are sure nothing has been added to the drink. Don't use the ice, since it may be from a contaminated source. Be careful not to swallow any water if you are swimming or showering. Swimming pools that are well chlorinated are probably safe.

How Can I Avoid Traveler's Diarrhea?

Since contaminated food and water can cause traveler's diarrhea, you need to be very careful of what you eat or drink. Choose restaurants that are well known or recommended by reliable people (hotel managers, coaches and athletes who have traveled in the area before). The U. S. Embassy is also a good place to get information about the restaurants and water conditions. Whenever you can, **avoid** food sold on the street corners or open air markets. Be very careful at buffets, especially outdoors. Make sure the hot foods that are served are hot and the cold foods cold.

You also need to be careful about the amount and type of food you eat while you are traveling. Try to keep your eating habits as close to normal as possible. If you don't usually eat fruit, don't over consume fruit while you travel. Eating too much of any food, even if it is a type of food you eat all the time, increases your chances of having diarrhea.

What Type of Foods Should I Eat?

Cooked foods are the best choice because the cooking process kills most organisms that can cause diarrhea. Well-cooked vegetables and meats that are well-done are good choices. Milk and milk products can be a little risky because they require pasteurization and complete re-frigeration. Milk products may be safe at first-class hotels. Also, fruits that can be peeled, like oranges, grapefruit, and bananas, are safer be-cause the part you eat is naturally protected by the skin. It is recom-mended that you peel the fruit yourself. Packing non-perishable foods from home help on those days where you are suspect of the food that is being served. Table 8.6 lists foods that travel well and are non-perish-able.

Table 8.6. Non-perishable foods for international travel.

Assorted cold cereals (individual packs)
Packets of instant oatmeal
Carnation instant breakfast
Fruit roll-ups
Kellogg's Nutrigrain bars
Peanut butter
Fruit juice
Breadsticks
Crackers (make sure that hydrogenated fat is not in the first two ingredients)
Graham crackers
Vanilla wafers
Fat-free fig newtons
Nonfat pretzels
Snackwell cookies
Canned tuna
Baked beans (look for the vegetarian or fat-free)
Dried fruit (raisins, apples, bananas, apricots, cranberry)
Microwave popcorn (select those that have less than 20% of the calories from fat)
Canned fruits (peaches and pears)

What Should I Do If I Have Traveler's Diarrhea?

If you should develop diarrhea, stop eating solid foods until the gas, cramps and stomach pains go away. If available, drink large amounts of a sport drink or fluid replacement drink with bottled water. Otherwise, try the **BRAT** diet, that is *B* for bananas; *R* for rice; *A* for applesauce; and *T* for toast. Those food are usually available no mat-ter what country you are traveling in, and they help with restoring muscle and liver glycogen. Carbonated beverages should be kept to a minimum. Try not to take medication which might stop the diarrhea. Your body is trying to get rid of the microbe that is causing the diar-rhea and taking medication may not enable the body to get rid of it. If the diarrhea persists for more than 48 hours, see a doctor.

GUIDELINES FOR EATING AT ALL-DAY EVENTS ⎯⎯⎯

Some athletic events such as swim meets, track meets, wrestling tournaments, volleyball tournaments, and tennis tournaments can last all day and competition may continue for several days. If you participate in a sport that lasts all day, you need to replenish carbohydrate stores and make sure you are well-hydrated for peak performance. It is also important that you eat after you compete to make sure that you will have enough energy in the muscles for the next day's competition.

The same diet principle used to plan the pre-game meal can also apply to foods eaten at all-day competition. If a swimmer races at 10:00 am and again in two hours, foods that are high in protein and fat will more than likely be in the swimmer's stomach causing some type of gastrointestinal distress as he get ready to race. The following guidelines have been recommended to help athletes make wise food choices at athletic events that last all day.

- If you have an hour or less between events or heats you should stick with carbohydrate foods that are in liquid form, such as juices and sport drinks. If you want something solid to eat, try fruits like oranges, peaches, pears, and bananas. These foods are mostly carbohydrates and water. They will be digested very fast and, therefore, will not cause as much of a problem with stomach cramping or GI distress. Another key point to making food choices with a limited time between competitions is to limit the amount of food you eat. The more you consume the longer it will take to digest, especially when you are nervous.

- If you have two to three hours between events or heats, you should add more solid carbohydrates like bagels, hot or cold cereal, English muffins along with some type of fruit like bananas, apples, oranges, and peaches. Make sure that you are still drinking fluids, like a sport drink, for rehydration and restoration of muscle glycogen.

- If you have four hours or more between events or heats, you can have basically a meal, but the meal should be composed primarily of carbohydrates. For example, a turkey sandwich on two slices of whole grain bread, low-fat yogurt with fruit and a sport drink or spaghetti with meat sauce, bread and sport drink are all appropriate. Remember, if you have a winning combination stick to it. Don't try a new combination of foods or different foods during the most important race of your life. Instead, try these new foods during training or a lesser competition to see if they are agreeable to you. Don't make eating between events and heats a dietary disaster by eating at the concession stand. Most concession stands are filled with high-fat, high-caloric foods that are not designed to maximize your performance. It is always wise to pack a cooler from home with winning combinations rather than to rely on a concession stand. Table 8.3 has a list of nutrient-dense, carbohydrate foods that are easy to pack in a cooler.

PUTTING IT ALL TOGETHER _____

Because athletes have a high requirement for carbohydrates and sometimes have a difficult time making wise food choices, they need to learn the following strategies on how to eat better while traveling to and from competitions. First, it is important to learn that the food guide pyramid can be used as a guide in making food decisions (see Chapter 4, Figure 4.5). Second, identify where you are going to eat and pay close attention to the type and amount of high-carbohydrate foods selected from restaurant menus. If the opportunity arises, try and take a nutrition class or summer course that will give you the skills and strategies to make wise food choices for athletic competition, as well as for the rest of your life. Last but not least, be a role model for the rest of the team and especially young athletes. Young children, participating in sport, emulate the behaviors of elite coaches and athletes. It makes no sense to stress the importance of good nutrition on athletic performance when a parent, role model athlete or coach is on the pool deck or sideline overconsuming coffee and eating doughnuts. We must educate young athletes so they have the knowledge to make wise food choices, and when the opportunity arises, set a good example.

Appendix A
Healthy Reading

INTRODUCTION

As we have seen there are three major physical variables in athletic performance — genetics, training and nutrition. Nothing can be done about the first. There are hundreds of books on the second; and the third is probably the most important, for as we have seen in the previous chapters it is the least understood. For all who exercise at any level, there are other books on the market that can serve as resources for additional information regarding nutrition and training. It is often difficult for athletes to distinguish between the reputable nutrition author and the self-proclaimed nutrition expert. Nutrition quacks often promote products based on unsubstantiated scientific claims. They try to establish their credibility by associating themselves with professional and amateur athletes. They generally promise superior health and performance. They rely heavily on testimonials and case histories to promote their product's effectiveness, and they typically find fault with an individual's eating habits.

THE DANGER

Nutrition quackery would not be a problem if all the advice were cheap and safe. Too often it is neither, and in some cases it can be life threatening. For example, potassium chloride, a substance often sold as a diet supplement, is potentially dangerous and overuse can be fatal.

Athletes who consume Chinese herbs and teas to enhance performance may find themselves eliminated from competition after drug testing. Herbs and herbal teas contain many different chemical compounds, some of which may be listed on the banned drug list. Amino acid supplements are often touted as being beneficial for strength because they claim to provide a safe anabolic or muscle building effect.

The amino acid arginine and ornithine are theorized to increase the levels of human growth hormone (hGH), which has a strong anabolic effect. Research has found that injections of large doses of amino acid arginine may cause the body to release greater amounts of growth hormone, however, the small amounts found in the food supplements do not increase levels of growth hormone or provide an anabolic effect. In fact, exercise itself normally promotes a much greater increase in growth hormone secretion than taking supplements. In addition, excess growth hormone does not increase athletic ability or help eliminate fat from the body. Instead it may lead to acromegaly, **which is characterized by disfiguring enlargements of the bones of the face, hands and feet.**

Food faddists may also convince healthy athletes to use popular fad diets to control weight and alter body composition. Many of these fad diets supply large amounts of saturated fat and cholesterol, which are associated with cardiovascular disease. The very low-calorie diets are not appropriate for athletes because they cannot meet the training needs and probably will promote loss of lean body mass and depletion of carbohydrate stores.

RELIABLE NUTRITION INFORMATION

It is easy to find books about nutrition. What is not so simple is evaluating these books to find one that is accurate and reliable. Before purchasing a nutrition and training resource, evaluate its credibility by reviewing the table of contents and asking the following questions:

- What credentials does the author have? What degrees does the author have, in what field, and from what institution? Many authors have letters behind their names but they are from unaccredited universities or diploma mills. The author may have never attended the university or taken a nutrition class. In 1985, a congressional panel estimated that 500,000 Americans possess fraudulent mail-order credentials or diploma-mill degrees. Nutrition is especially fertile as an arena for fraud.
- Is the author a member of a reputable organization? Professional organizations can be researched in the library to see who belongs to this group, how many members do they have, and is their board elected on a regular basis.
- Does the author promote eating a wide variety of foods or does he/she improperly recommend the elimination of certain food groups? Eliminating any one of the five food groups will lead to deficiencies and decreased performance.

- Does the author recommend relying on foods or using large amounts of supplements to obtain nutrients? Quacks often rely upon the incorrect concept that you cannot get all the nutrients you need out of the food supply. They claim that in order to improve performance or health you must purchase their products.
- Is the information factual and specific or vague and highly emotional? They generally tell you all the wonderful things that their products can do in your body and/or all the horrible things that can happen if you don't get enough. But they conveniently neglect to tell you that a balanced diet can provide all the nutrients you need, and the Food Guide Pyramid system makes balancing your diet simple.
- Are the recommendations based on scientific evidence or on personal testimonials and anecdotes? We all tend to believe what others tell us about personal experiences. But separating cause and effect from coincidence can be difficult. If people tell you that product X has cured their cancer, arthritis, or whatever, be skeptical. They may have never had the condition. If they did, their recovery most likely would have occurred without the help of product X. Establishing medical truths requires careful and repeated investigations — with well-designed experiments, not reports of misperceived cause and effect.
- Does the author seem to agree with most recommendations from medical, sports science and nutrition professionals? Quacks, who want you to trust them, suggest that most health professionals are "butchers and poisoners." Credible professionals rely upon sound, scientific principles. These principles are founded in courses such as nutrition, biochemistry, and physiology. All these courses are required in every medical school as well as academic schools that train sports scientists and nutrition professionals.

DISTINGUISHING A SPORTS NUTRITIONIST FROM A FADDIST

How can athletes choose a reliable source for sports nutrition? A reputable sports nutritionist should:

- individualize a diet plan for each athlete's unique needs that is based on lifestyle and medical history
- consult with the team or athlete's physician and/or sports scientist if the athlete is under treatment
- encourage meeting dietary requirements through eating a wide variety of foods instead of relying on vitamin and mineral supplements

- recommend limiting weight loss for athletes to 1-3 pounds per week
- advise that health and performance depend on many factors, nutrition being only one.

A responsible, qualified sports nutritionist should **not:**

- promise miraculous improvements in performance or muscular strength
- claim that everyone needs nutrient supplements or health foods
- use pseudomedical jargon such as "detoxifying your body," "balancing your chemistry," "strengthening your immune system," or "oxygenating your blood"
- promise quick, easy, or dramatic weight loss or cures
- sell nutrient supplements after recommending them to an athlete.

Combating nutrition quackery is no easy task. Parents, coaches, and athletes need to critically evaluate nutrition claims and products, and learn to ask specific questions. If fraud is suspected, they may wish to contact law enforcement agencies, legislators, physicians, reputable nutritionists, exercise physiologists or nutrition organizations. The best weapon against nutrition misinformation is the dissemination of sound, credible information.

RECOMMENDED SOURCES ⎯⎯⎯⎯⎯

Here are some additional books and newsletters that will guide you to a path of good nutrition and improved performance. While there are numerous nutrition and diet books on the market, there are only a few available that are written for active individuals, without a Ph.D. in nutrition. Here are a few of our favorites that will give you straight answers to your questions and nutritional needs.

Books

The Really Simple No Nonsense Nutrition Guide
Edward R. Blonz, Ph.D.
Conari Press, Berkeley, CA, 1993

Blonz, a syndicated nutrition and health columnist, presents straight answers to nutrition questions. The book contains many easy-to-read tables and figures, and he writes in a very informal style to help you learn everything you wanted to know about diet food and your health. There are chapters on how to shop at the supermarket, and he wraps up the book with a chapter on how to construct a simple, no nonsense eating plan.

Eating on the Run
Evelyn Tribole, MS, RD
Leisure Press, Champaign, IL, 1992

Eating on the Run gives you nutritional information needed to make healthy eating choices and beat the clock. Do you know how to make the healthiest choices at McDonald's? How can you squeeze healthy, nutritious meals into your busy schedule. Includes 40 mini meals that take just one minute to fix; advice on coping with power meals and happy hour worries; tips on how to avoid the fat traps in healthy sounding convenient foods; snacks for your gym bag; and detailed information on 400-plus fast foods.

Nancy Clark's Sports Nutrition Guidebook
Nancy Clark, MS, RD
Leisure Press, Champaign, IL, 1990

This book helps you create a winning diet for high energy and lifelong health. But you won't have to spend hours in the kitchen, give up eating out or totally avoid fast foods. This book contains over 100 fast, practical and nutritious recipes that are ideal for an athlete's sports diet.

Eating for Endurance
Ellen Coleman, MA, MPH, RD
Bull Publishing Company, Palo Alto, CA, 1989

Throughout her book, Ellen Coleman addresses the everyday needs of those who exercise for health, or just to improve their body image, as well as the needs of elite athletes who want to shave minutes or seconds off their competitive times. For all who exercise at any level, this book can help them excel, stay healthy, and enjoy the athletic performance.

Power Foods
Liz Applegate, Ph.D.
Rodale Press, Emmaus, PA, 1991

Not just for athletes, this book is an excellent guide to good nutrition for all of us. Chock full of tips on how to incorporate healthy eating into any lifestyle. Gives useful tips on how to gauge the impact of your vitamin and mineral level on everyday performance. You'll also find out how to feast on fast foods and still save on calories and fat. *Power Foods* features scores of quick reference charts and lists that spotlight the nutritional best in snacks, beverages, breakfast cereals, fast food fare, and even sweets.

Food For Sport
Nathan J. Smith, MD, and Bonnie Worthington-Roberts, Ph.D.
Bull Publishing Company, Palo Alto, CA, 1989

This book is about food — what it is and what it does, and how it can be chosen selectively to maximize physical performance. This book is directed to a wide range of readers: the casual sports participant to the highly skilled athlete. It provides basic information that will enhance your understanding of the nutritional needs of various sports so you can achieve a better level of athletic performance . . . and lifelong health.

Outsmarting the Female Fat Cell
Debra Waterhouse, MPH, RD
Hyperion Books, New York

The first weight control program designed specifically for women. Highly acclaimed from the moment it was published, this innovative book tells you why the female fat cell thrives on diets and shows the effects of estrogen, oral contraceptives, pregnancy, menopause and hormone replacement therapy on fat storage. Break the endless diet cycle and begin a new, natural sensible way of eating that feeds your body, not your fat cell.

The Tufts University Guide to Total Nutrition
Stanley Gershoff, M.D.
Harper and Row, New York, 1990

This comprehensive and up-to-date volume by the dean of the prestigious Tufts University School of Nutrition is written in a style that makes it particularly easy to read and use. An introductory section on nutrition fundamentals is followed by sections that deal with the American diet, nutritional life-styles, the diet-health connection, and keeping fit and trim. Based on the latest nutrition findings, this book features a series of nutrition quizzes and contains many practical suggestions for eating better.

Newsletters

Tufts University Diet and Nutrition Letter
P.O. Box 57857
Boulder, CO 80322-7857
800-274-7581

Nutrition Action Healthletter
Center for Science in the Public Interest
1875 Connecticut Ave. N W, Suite 300
Washington, DC 20009-5728
202-332-9110

Harvard Medical School Health Letter
Department of Continuing Education
25 Shattuck St.
Boston, MA 02115

Sports Medicine Digest
P.O. Box 2468
Van Nuys, CA 91404

Mayo Clinic Nutrition Letter
200 1st Street SW
Rochester, MN 55905
1-800-888-3968

University of California Berkeley Wellness Letter
P.O. Box 420148
Palm Coast, FL 32142

Periodicals

American Health Magazine: Fitness of Body and Mind
P.O. Box 3015
Harlan, IA 51537-3015

Cooking Light Magazine
P.O. Box C-549
Birmingham, AL 35283

In Health Magazine
P.O. Box 52431
Boulder, CO 80320-2431

Hotlines

American Diabetes Association
1-800-ADA-DISC

Bulimia Anorexia Self-Help
1-800-227-4785

National Health Information Center
1-800-336-4797
(in MD call 301-656-4167)

Local Resources

- Cooperative extension agents in county extension offices.
- State list of Consulting Dietitians. The American Dietetic Association will send you a list of consulting R.D.'s in your state. Send a self-addressed, stamped envelope to Nutrition Resources Department, American Dietetic Association, 216 West Jackson Blvd., Suite 800, Chicago, IL 60606-6995.
- Nutrition faculty and/or exercise science faculty affiliated with departments of food and nutrition, sports science, or kinesiology at your local university or college.
- Exercise Physiologists contact the American College of Sports Medicine, 401 West Michigan Street, Indianapolis, IN 46202 (317-637-9200).

Appendix B
Nutritional Software

Like to keep track of your calories consumed and the amount of protein in your diet, but hate trying to determine how many grams of protein, carbohydrate and fat are in every portion of food you eat? If so, you might want to invest in nutrition software for your computer. The better nutrition programs are easy to install, easy to use and surprisingly affordable. And once you are up to speed on them, they can be a lot of fun and provide valuable information for your training log.

No matter what type of nutritional software you plan to use, you must have the appropriate hardware. Different software programs will require different amounts of memory and some are not made for the Macintosh. Make sure you read the package and sales information as each software package has different requirements.

The only problem with comparing computerized nutrition programs is that it is a lot like comparing apples and oranges—both are fruits, high in simple sugars and low in fat, but they come in very different packages. Likewise, nutrition software are similar in many ways, but the way they report information and the way they present it are sometimes very different.

The software below was judged on what information was provided in their manuals, how well they provide the information, and how easy the programs are to use on your home computer. With these caveats in mind, nutritional software can be a worthwhile investment of your time and money if you are serious about proper nutrition and its affect on your performance.

Here are some of the "Home" versions of nutrition (some also contain exercise files) software on the market.

The Diet Balancer ($59.95)
Nutridata Software Corporation
PO Box 769
1215 Route 9, Ste. F
Wappingers Falls, NY 12590
800-922-2988

Ranks foods as "low" or "high" by nutrients; allows you to include your vitamin supplements (most programs do not have this feature); plots your weight for up to two months; charts your weekly and monthly nutrient averages. Some important ingredients such as baking soda (if one is on a low sodium diet) is missing, some foods are listed in grams and not ounces, and no data is included on beta carotene or chromium.

Perfect Diet ($49.00)
1142 Old Boalsburg Road
State College, PA 16801
800-852-8446

Lets you develop realistic weight loss programs, then charts them for up to six months. It analyzes your diet for 27 nutrients and tracks nutrient intake for a day, week, month or quarter. You can add foods to database or enter recipes, and it will analyze the food for you. Program can track up to nine individuals at once. Some people find that the large number of options make it cumbersome to use.

DINE Healthy ($99.00)
DINE Systems, Inc.
586 North French Road, Ste. 2
Amherst, NY, 14228
800-688-1848

The user-expandable database contains over 7000 foods analyzed for 26 nutrients. You can also look up foods individually by common name, brand name, or nickname. You can sort your food selections by nutrients for an in-depth look at sources and amounts. DINE Healthy highlights potential diet problems for quick and easy food exchanges. DINE Healthy helps you design a weight control program that works. Track your progress on a daily, weekly, and monthly basis. The program provides weight loss/gain charts to help you monitor your progress in controlling your weight.

Nutrition Pro ($29 for home version, $79 for professional version)
ESHA Research
PO Box 13028
Salem, OR 97309
503-585-6242

A very complete and comprehensive program. It contains 2,000 foods and you can add up to 50 new foods. It records personal statistics, exercise activities, and foods consumed are easy to enter. It will calculate your individual daily requirements based on the RDA, analyze dietary intake and identify deficiencies or excesses. It will store data for up to ten individuals. Portion sizes are realistic, and you can design a daily menu to meet your daily nutrient and caloric needs. Only analyzes your diet for 16 nutrients and does not include such nutrients as chromium, folic acid and zinc.

UltraCoach ($59.95)
9635 Monte Vista Ave.
Suite 201
Montclair, CA 91763-2235
800-400-1390

If you are a runner, cyclist or swimmer, UltraCoach wants to be your personal trainer. Enter information about your exercise habits and goals, and the software gives you a five week workout routine. The program also tracks your daily caloric intake and output, determines your target heart rate during workouts, recommends the pace at which you should exercise and lets you print graphs of your progress and health status.

Here are the Cadillac versions that have very extensive databases and are more applicable for team use:

Food Processor ($295 basic version, $495 for plus version)
ESHA Research
PO Box 13028
Salem, OR 97309
503-585-6242

The big brother version of Nutrition Pro, does about everything, even plans menus and helps you reach your fat and caloric goals. It has a data base of over 3,000 foods and analyzes your diet for 49 nutrients, the Plus, 105 nutrients. Food Processor features 75 functions for nutrient analysis and menu planning, including individual nutrition information, single nutrient analysis, and average analysis over time. Will even give analysis of amino-acid content of foods.

Nutritionist IV Diet Analysis ($495)
N-Squared Computing
First DataBank Division
The Hearst Corp.
1111 Bayhill Drive, Suite 270,
San Bruno, CA 94066
800-289-1701

One of the most complete and comprehensive programs of those that we reviewed. It analyzes your diet for over 75 nutrients and tells you what percentage of your goal you have consumed, based upon a questionnaire you fill out when first using the program. The database has over 12,000 different foods, which include brand names, fast foods, and ethnic foods. Entry of food and diet information is very easy, and the program also has the ability to generate weight-loss or weight-gain profiles, including diet and exercise information and activity schedules.

Also included with the software package is the FIT III program, which creates exercise programs, progress reports and information on how much energy you have expended — a great feature for active individuals. Expect to spend over 15 minutes to do a complete analysis of your daily diet.

Appendix C
Your Guide To Label-Ease™

When you see the words "Nutrition Facts," you know you're reading a new food label. Here are some tips for using food labels to help you choose healthful foods.

Check the serving size and servings per container to see how they compare to your usual serving of the food.

Fat is only one concern in a healthful diet. Make sure the foods you pick also provide fiber, vitamins and minerals – the health protectors in food.

The sugars on this line can be naturally occuring ones – like the carbohydrates found in milk (lactose) or fruit (fructose) or simple sugars added during processing of foods (baked goods and mixes, cereals, beverages, etc.). Check the ingredient label to identify which types of sugars are in a food item.

Nutrition Facts

Serving Size 1 cup (228g)
Servings Per Container 2

Amount Per Serving

Calories 260   Calories from Fat 120

	% Daily Value*
Total Fat 13g	**20%**
Saturated Fat 5g	**25%**
Cholesterol 30mg	**10%**
Sodium 660mg	**28%**
Total Carbohydrate 31g	**10%**
Dietary Fiber 0g	**0%**
Sugars 5g	
Protein 5g	

Vitamin A 4%	•	Vitamin C 2%	
Calcium 15%	•	Iron 4%	

* Percent Daily Values are based on a 2,000 calorie diet. Your daily values may be higher or lower depending on your calorie needs:

	Calories:	2,000	2,500
Total Fat	Less than	65g	80g
Sat Fat	Less than	20g	25g
Cholesterol	Less than	300mg	300mg
Sodium	Less than	2,400mg	2,400mg
Total Carbohydrate		300g	375g
Dietary Fiber		25g	30g

Calories per gram:
Fat 9 • Carbohydrate 4 • Protein 4

The % Daily Value gives a general idea of a food's nutrient contributions to a 2,000 calorie reference diet.

% Daily Value for Fat shows how the amount of fat in a serving of this food compares to 65 grams, the Daily Value for fat for a 2,000 calorie reference diet. It does not mean percent calories from fat for this food.

These are the nutrient pluses in foods. Most Americans need more of these vitamins, minerals and fiber. A value of 10% or more means the food is a good source of that nutrient.

This reference chart appears the same on all food labels that carry it.

157

Words You Can Trust

Label terms and descriptors such as "low fat," "low sodium," "high," "reduced," etc., are now legally defined for food companies. These terms are standard across all brands and types of foods. For example, you can trust that "low sodium" on a label means the food, in the labeled portion size, meets the criteria for low sodium foods.

Health Claims

Food labels can now carry a claim about how a food or nutrient in a food can lessen the risk of certain diseases. All health claims must follow specific guidelines. For example, foods high in calcium, such as milk, can say:

"Regular exercise and a healthy diet with enough calcium help teen and young adult white and Asian women maintain good bone health and may reduce their high risk for osteoporosis later in life."

Currently there are 7 health claims approved for use on food labels.

Five Tips For Using The New Food Label

1. Compare similar foods such as soup to soup, cereal to cereal, yogurt to yogurt. Comparing like products will help you determine which one is the best buy for your nutrition needs.
2. Most people have **similar** fiber, vitamin and mineral needs while most people have **different** calorie needs. Calories determine the Daily Values for protein, carbohydrate and fat. The label lists Daily Values for someone who needs 2,000 calories a day. Your calorie needs may be either higher or lower.
3. Healthful diets are based on food patterns over time. Eat a variety of foods from each of the five food groups — milk, fruit, vegetable, meat, grains — each day. Use food labels to help make choices within a food group to meet your health and taste preferences.
4. Any food can fit in a healthful diet. Reading labels can help you balance choices and enjoy your favorite foods.
5. To learn more about label reading, contact a registered dietitian (RD) or certified home economist (CHE) at your local medical center, health department or extension office. For group programs, the Label Ease videotape program on using the new labels is available for loan from Idaho Dairy Council, 1365 N. Orchard, Suite 203, Boise, ID 83706.

Source: *Label Facts for Healthful Eating*, Browne, Mona B., National Food Processors Association, 1993.
©Idaho Dairy Council, 1994.

Index